PSYCHIATRY - THEORY, APPLICATIONS AND TREATMENTS

HUMANIST PSYCHIATRY

2ND EDITION

Psychiatry - Theory, Applications and Treatments

Additional books and e-books in this series can be found on Nova's website under the Series tab.

PSYCHIATRY - THEORY, APPLICATIONS AND TREATMENTS

HUMANIST PSYCHIATRY

2ND EDITION

NASH N. BOUTROS, MD

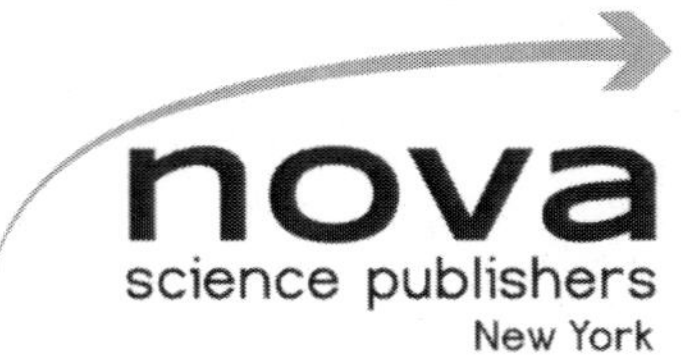

DOI: https://doi.org/10.52305/UHDH1142

NOTICE TO THE READER

Library of Congress Cataloging-in-Publication Data

Names: Boutros, Nashaat N., author.
Title: Humanist psychiatry / Nash N. Boutros.
Description: 2nd edition. | New York : Nova Science Publishers, [2022] | Series: Psychiatry - theory, applications and treatments | Includes bibliographical references and index. |
Identifiers: LCCN 2021062779 (print) | LCCN 2021062780 (ebook) | ISBN 9781685075019 (paperback) | ISBN 9781685075446 (adobe pdf)
Subjects: LCSH: Psychiatry.
Classification: LCC RC454 .B67 2022 (print) | LCC RC454 (ebook) | DDC 616.89--dc23/eng/20211230
LC record available at https://lccn.loc.gov/2021062779
LC ebook record available at https://lccn.loc.gov/2021062780

Published by Nova Science Publishers, Inc. † New York

Contents

PREFACE

This book is an outcry for all who care about human suffering in any form but particularly in the form of psychiatric disorders. The principle of worth and dignity does not place a price, nor takes into consideration, the cost of taking care of human beings. The fact of the matter is that it is the budget for "mental health" that gets chopped off when money is short. The budgets for psychiatric care are minimal compared to budgets for other disorders. Without a strong grass root movement to propel research and advocacy for psychiatric care, the current status is likely to remain unchanged with suffering continuing inside long-term psychiatric care facilities, community mental health centers, and even in the most affluent psychiatric care facilities. As will be argued in the chapter "Integrated System" the future of the practice of psychiatry is likely to be both expensive and highly effective. According to humanist principles, the high cost of effective care should never be allowed to be an obstacle or excuse for not making all possible resources fully available to an individual patient.

This book is not about the practice of psychiatry but rather about how the field is conceptualized, organized, and propelled forward. Despite the huge advances in the neurosciences in the last 30 to 40 years, the practice of psychiatry has remained stagnant except for few newer and safer medications. When I practiced psychiatry in Cairo or rural Egypt in the mid-seventies the main diagnostic method was asking patients about their past and current experiences, an almost completely subjective system of assessment. This remains exactly the same today.

The most important aspect of this book is how to view psychiatry from a Humanist viewpoint with the scientific method, human worth and dignity and the democratic process. When data from literature are discussed, they are never meant to be exhaustive reviews. The literature is marshaled to support a point and is simplified for the non-professional reader. The opposing point, if there is one, is frequently not discussed in similar detail.

Psychiatric disorders remain devastatingly widespread, under-recognized and under-treated worldwide. Psychiatric disorders are among the most common causes for disability and lost productivity. Psychiatric patients have shorter lives - 15-20 years less than mentally healthy populations. A British study by the Health Economics Research Group suggested that for every pound spent on psychiatric research the economy regained 37 pence per year in benefits from increased productivity, and reduced health care bills. This is about the same rate of return on cardiovascular research expenditures (The Economist October 24th, 2015).

While the brain by itself is immensely complex and its constant interactions with other bodily systems, like the neuroendocrine and metabolic systems, compound the complexity, the interaction between the brain and the environment remains one of the largest scientific conquests. Nonetheless, all the advances in neuroscience research clearly and overwhelmingly point to the eventual unraveling of the mysteries of this organ. We, in psychiatry, cannot wait the decades it will take to fully understand the brain. Neuroscience research has already given us much insight into many disorders. We are, in fact, at a stage where it will be very hard for anyone to argue that schizophrenia, bipolar disorder or obsessive-compulsive disorder (OCD) are not biological phenomena reflecting various forms of brain dysfunction. Some other, and equally devastating disorders, are not yet so fortunate. Strikingly, I have attended many meetings where social anxiety or addiction disorders are discussed in purely non-neuroscience language. This simply reflects the lack of significant neuroscience research in these disorders as well as the lack of dissemination of the available findings to the psychiatric community and to patients and their families. The National Institutes of Mental Health (NIMH) has indicated its support for the concept that ALL psychiatric disorders are in fact neurocircuitry disturbances.

Advocacy for the psychiatrically ill is also extremely weak. Given the prevalence of psychiatric disorders (It is estimated one out of five humans suffer from one or more), a well organized advocacy organization not unlike the National Rifle Association (NRA) or the American Association for Retired Persons (AARP), would indeed be very influential. Factoring in family members of psychiatric patients, all those who care for these patients as well as all activists in this field, I can see such organization to surpass all other advocacy organizations combined in its ability to enhance the rate of advancement in this field.

The issue of stigma is also well recognized. Efforts to combat the stigma associated with receiving any psychiatric diagnosis or even just seeing a psychiatrist are many but have met with hardly any progress. The recalcitrant nature of the "mental illness" stigma will remain as long as the term "mental" remains. These disorders are stigmatizing because they are "mental" as opposed to regular physical disorders.

As will be repeatedly argued throughout this volume, our way out of stigma must go through the brain. I am amazed that in a recent article entitled "Fighting the stigma caused by mental disorders: past perspectives, present activities, and future directions" there was no mention of the brain, psychiatric disorders as brain disorders or neuroscience in general (Stuart, 2008). "Epilepsy" for as long as its brain etiology was unknown, was a highly stigmatizing disorder. This is hardly the case now. The term "mental" embodies the duality of mind-brain or mental-physical. Doing away with this duality is our first step to burying stigma and relegating it to history of medicine.

ACKNOWLEDGMENTS

Without the constant support of my wife (Sylvia) and my children (Tammer and Alexandria), I could not have been able to complete this edition of "Humanist Psychiatry." I also would like to acknowledge all my colleagues who commented on the first edition. Those comments were taken to heart in preparing the current edition. I would also like to acknowledge Linda Cashdan for the thorough professional editing of the book. Finally, I would like to express my utmost gratitude to Alexandria Boutros for her significant contribution to the "Correctional Psychiatry" chapter.

Introduction to the Second Edition

Since the publication of the first edition of *Humanist Psychiatry*, I received significant feedback mainly reflecting the desire of many mental-health professionals who are not MDs or PhDs to have access to the book. In response, I have simplified the language and rearranged the flow for easier accessibility to all mental-health professionals including social workers, case managers and therapists.

Humanism is an optimistic philosophy that believes in two major tenets. The first is that no matter how difficult a problem is, the human brainpower, as demonstrated over the history of humankind, is capable of solving it. It is a matter of whether there is the desire to solve it. Once the desire is there (as in the current desire to cure cancer), it becomes a matter of resources and time.

The second major tenet is that every human deserves the best possible life. It is from both principles that the concepts of Humanist Psychiatry flow. As will be described in the following chapters, no ailment should be considered part of nature, and as such, acceptable as part of a spectrum. Each human deserves a full chance on life. This idea necessitates the dedication of resources not only to research causes and treatments of the various psychiatric disorders but also to the necessary resources for the *primary prevention* of the disorders when risk factors are already known. NO ONE HAS THE RIGHT TO SAVE MONEY BY

NOT PROVIDING ALL POSSIBLE RESOURCES TO PREVENT THE ILLNESS FROM OCCURING OR AMELIORATING THE EFFECTS ONCE IT DOES.

How Did I Come to Subscribe to Humanism?

I was born in a highly religious family environment. As a Middle-Eastern Christian the major concept was that everything that happens is pre-determined. A higher power determines who gets ill and who wins a lottery. At age eleven, I had two younger sisters and two older brothers. We were a church-going family steeped in Coptic Orthodoxy. One of my two beloved sisters contracted TB-Meningitis. Despite the best care available in 1950s Egypt, she suffered a great deal and eventually died. I simply could not understand why this should happen to anyone. The answer I was given by my family (and the community) was that that was GOD's will. This answer simply raised more questions than it answered. Why would GOD, presumably benevolent, allow this immense suffering to occur to an absolutely innocent person as well as to her, also innocent family, including myself?

While I could not help the questioning in my mind, there was no way to voice these doubts out loud. Some light became available when one of my older brothers began allowing me to read his "existentialism" books. He acquired those books in order to be masterful in arguing against anyone who dared to question the prevailing wisdom by citing these books with their famous authors like Jan Paul Sartre, Georg Hegel or Søren Kierkegaard. In fact, they had quite the opposite effect on my questioning and indeed agonizing mind.

Once in medical school I started learning about diseases and their causation. In my wanderings through the huge facilities of the Kasr-El-Eini Cairo University Faculty of Medicine, I found myself in the pediatric oncology ward. I have never experienced such horror. The ward was full of children little and big, boys and girls, all with IVs and eyes looking out at me with utter despair. Undoubtedly, many of them had not yet realized the sentences they were handed; and in the mid-sixties those were mainly death sentences. Parents on the other hand new what lay ahead. It became so utterly clear to me that GOD was the absolute only hope they had to overcome this horrendous outlook. Indeed, if GOD did not exist, they had no option but to invent him. The doctors were as helpless as the patients were. Nevertheless, many of the doctors subscribed to the notion that this was GOD's will and that we simply had to resign to it. I heard the Docs repeatedly feed this line to the families. I never once heard a doctor tell a family that we simply do not know how to treat this ailment and that we are sorry that science has not gotten us there yet. Of course, that would not nearly be as comforting as stating that miracles do happen and we should hope for one! My issue here is not with what the doctors told the patients to comfort them (which is reasonable) but in what they themselves believed in.

Reading about the horrors of the black plague, cholera and tuberculosis (which is actually what killed her), and how medical advances could completely eliminate these ailments, I had no doubt in mind that if medical science available to Egyptian doctors back then was at the level it is today where TB is readily diagnosable and treatable, my beloved sister, Nadia, would not have had to die.

I thus am dedicating this book to her memory.

Chapter 1

HUMANISM PRICIPLES RELEVANT TO PSYCHIATRIC CARE

Humanism is optimistic regarding human nature and confident in human reason and science as the best means of reaching the goal of human fulfillment in this world. Humanists affirm that humans are a product of the same evolutionary process that produced all other organisms and that all ideas, knowledge, values, and social systems are based upon human experience. Humanists conclude that creative ability and personal responsibility are strongest when the mind is free from supernatural beliefs and operates in an atmosphere of freedom and democracy.

The following is a description of the humanist principles that pertain to the subject matter of this book, "Clinical Psychiatry." These principles were first published in the "Humanist" in the September/October issue of 1973 by the American Humanist Association in *Humanist Manifesto II.*

The *Humanist Manifesto* affirms that "Modern science discredits such historic concepts as the "ghost in the machine" and the "separable soul." Rather, science affirms that the human species is an emergence from natural evolutionary forces. As far as we know, the total personality is a function of the biological organism transacting in a social and cultural context. As originally stated in Humanist Manifesto I, published by the American Humanist Association 1933, “Humanists hold an organic view of life and affirm that the traditional dualism of mind and body must be rejected.”

The above principle is crucial for understanding human behavior and the nature of deviation in psychopathological conditions. Most importantly, this principle is important for deciding where to concentrate research dollars and efforts.

The next humanist principle with relevance to Clinical Psychiatry pertains to the value of the individual. The *Manifesto* affirms that, "The preciousness and dignity of the individual person is a central humanist value. Individuals should be encouraged to realize their own creative talents and desires. Humanism rejects all religious, ideological, or moral codes that denigrate the individual, suppress freedom, dull intellect, or dehumanize personality. Humanists believe in maximum individual autonomy consonant with social responsibility. Although science can account for the causes of behavior, the possibilities of freedom of choice exist in human life and should be increased.”

This principle affirms the supreme value of the individual human life and the supreme value placed by Humanism on the need to expend all efforts in assuring and helping individuals (particularly less fortunate ones) to realize their maximum potential and enjoy life to the fullest extent possible. This applies directly to the topic of this book as psychiatric disorders tend to rob their victims of autonomy, dignity, and the ability to enjoy life to the fullest.

The Humanist Principle of “Reason and Intelligence.” states that reason and intelligence are the most effective instruments that human kind possesses. There is no other substitute: neither faith nor passion suffices in itself. The controlled use of scientific methods, which have transformed the natural and social sciences since the Renaissance, must be extended further in the solution of human problems. But reason must be tempered with humility, since no group has a monopoly on wisdom or virtue. Nor is there any guarantee that all problems can be solved or all questions answered. Yet critical intelligence, infused by a sense of human caring, is the best method that humanity has for resolving problems.

Reason should be balanced with compassion and empathy. Thus, Humanism does not advocate the use of scientific intelligence independent of or in opposition to emotion, for Humanism believes in the cultivation of feeling and love. As science continually pushes out the boundary of the known and pushes back the boundaries of the unknown, humankind's sense of wonder is continually renewed.

The principle of "Reason and Intelligence" as the only method for increasing our knowledge is crucial for the future of psychiatry and how fast knowledge adequate to relieve the immense suffering, and better yet, to prevent it altogether, will be acquired. I would like to emphasize that there are no contradictions between the scientific method and anecdotal observations and intelligent, experience-based intuitions. Nonetheless, these must be considered only as starting points that should lead eventually to the full application of sound investigative methodologies. Reason and intelligence are the way out of blind research alleys. A blind research ally is created when passion or beliefs help to propel investigations that repeatedly lead nowhere.

On the other hand, reason and intelligence must be applied to the myriad of loose research ends that exist everywhere in psychiatric research. A loose end is created when an investigation uncovers an interesting and potentially useful finding but for some reason or the other the research effort comes to an end. The most frequent causes for this unfortunate outcome (which again is not uncommon) is loss of funding or loss of interest on part of the investigator. Here comes the absolute need for the practitioners to be aware of such findings and help propel the field from within and in a bottom-up fashion.

The *Humanist Principle* addressing human sexuality is also important for the practice of psychiatry. In the area of sexuality, Humanism proposes that intolerant attitudes, often cultivated by orthodox traditions and puritanical cultures, unduly repress sexual conduct. The right to birth control, abortion, and divorce should be recognized. While Humanism does not approve of exploitative, denigrating forms of sexual expression, neither does Humanism wish to prohibit, by law or social sanction, sexual behavior between consenting adults. The many varieties of sexual exploration should not in themselves be considered "wrong." Without countenancing mindless permissiveness or unbridled promiscuity, a civilized society should be a tolerant one. Short of harming others or compelling them to do likewise, individuals should be permitted to express their sexual proclivities and pursue their life styles as they desire. Humanism wishes to cultivate the development of a responsible attitude towards sexuality, in which humans are not exploited as sexual objects, and in which intimacy, sensitivity, respect, and honesty in interpersonal relationships are encouraged. Moral education for children and adults is an important way to developing awareness and sexual maturity.

The next impactful Humanist Principle pertains to the democratic ideal. Humanism strives to enhance freedom and dignity by assuring that individuals can experience a full range of civil liberties. Humanism, in fact, affirms the need to extend participatory democracy to all aspects of society. The conditions of work, education, devotion, and play should be humanized. Alienating forces should be modified or eradicated and bureaucratic structures should be held to a minimum. People are more important than decalogues, rules, proscriptions, or regulations. This principle may be most important to the governance of psychiatric institutions and academic departments of psychiatry.

An important principle pertains to moral equality. Moral equality should be furthered through the elimination of all discrimination based upon race, religion, sex, national origin, or age. This means equality of opportunity and recognition of talent.

This principle is of particular importance to psychiatry as many of the disorders may be related to conditions during pregnancy, delivery, early infancy and childhood. Drug use, malnutrition, and childhood or elderly abuse are all strongly related to socioeconomic factors.

The last two principles that pertain to our purpose relate to technological advances and globalization. First, we talk about technology. Humanism affirms that technology is a vital key to human progress and development. Humanism deplores any neo-romantic efforts to indiscriminately condemn all technology and science or to counsel retreat from its further extension and use for the good of humankind.

Humanism deplores any moves to censor basic scientific research on moral, political, or social grounds. Technology must, however, be carefully judged by the consequences of its use; harmful and destructive changes should be avoided. Humanism specifically deplores technological or bureaucratic control, manipulation, or modifying human beings without their fully-informed consent.

This principle is of particular significance and sensitivity since the fields of human genetic engineering and the advancing technologies that are capable of predicting future diseases while the human organism still evolving in the womb are rapidly evolving.

The final Principle to be discussed here is "Globalization." The problem of economic growth and development can no longer be resolved by one nation alone; it is worldwide in scope. In no place is this more necessary than in medicine in general and psychiatry in particular. Medical problems, including psychiatric disorders are human disorders with hardly any influence of culture. The prevalence of schizophrenia seems to be the same in both liberal and restrictive societies. Hence efforts at eradicating diseases should be worldwide efforts with international planning and cooperation.

Humanist psychiatry is based on the following four general principles:

1. That every effort should be made to alleviate the suffering of humans afflicted with psychiatric disorders. This includes providing best treatment available now and maximizing the scientific search for further understanding and treating of psychiatric disorders.
2. That our knowledge of the causes and treatments of psychiatric disorders remains minimal as evidenced by the lack of any proven etiology of any of the diseases included in the *Diagnostic and Statistical Manual (DSM)* published by the American Psychiatric Association and now in its fifth edition (DSM-5). Moreover, while many of the symptoms of psychiatric disorders

can be temporarily brought under control, no known cure exits for any of these disorders.

3. The third principle is that advancing knowledge regarding the brain, its physiology, anatomy, chemistry, genetics, and the impact of social interactions (including trauma and abuse) on all these areas is essential for the eventual understanding and effective treatment of such disorders.
4. The final principle is that all disorders are considered biological in origin until proven otherwise. This is in total opposition to current attitudes where if there is no readily apparent biological correlate the disorder is considered "psychological" or a disorder of the mind and not the brain. The best current example is personality disorders and to some extent addictive disorders.

Chapter 2

THE BIOLOGY PRINCIPLE

We must recollect that all our provisional ideas in psychology will presumably one day be based on an organic substructure.
Sigmund Freud

The separation of psychology from the premises of biology is purely artificial, because the human psyche lives in indissoluble union with the body.
C. G. Jung

Men ought to know that from the brain, and from the brain only, arise our pleasures, joys, laughter, and jests, as well as our sorrows, pains, grief, and fears. Through it, in particular, we think, see, hear... –
Hippocrates

In "On the Sacred Disease" Hippocrates disparages the notion that seizures arise from magical or demonic interference with life's processes (Jones 1923 and Grensemann 1968). Instead, the occurrence of seizures and other abnormalities are unequivocally attributed to the occurrence of disturbance of "natural" processes in the brain. It is the same thing that makes us mad or delirious, inspires us with dread and fear, aimless anxieties, absent-mindedness, and acts that are contrary to habit. These things that we suffer all come from the brain, when it is not healthy, but becomes abnormally hot, cold, moist or dry. Madness comes from its moistness. When the brain is abnormally moist, of necessity it moves, and when it moves, neither sight nor hearing is still, but we see or hear now one thing and now another, and the tongue speaks in accordance with the things seen and heard on each occasion (Grensemann 1968).

The Biology Principle dictates that persistent psychiatric deviations must be rooted in some form of biological brain abnormality. While it is entirely possible that faulty information can lead to faulty behavior, the brain has very powerful mechanisms that allow it to learn what behavior is advantageous and what is not and correct the output accordingly. Furthermore, the brain has a rather strong capacity for checking reality and correcting its world view to arrive at the most advantageous view of the world in the individual's particular circumstances. All these mechanisms require major brain systems that need to be intact to function properly.

Let's briefly talk about the brain. It is mainly composed of cells called "neurons." Each one of these cells is a computer. The brain has between 50 and 100 billion neurons. They communicate with each other in two different ways; either directly through what are called "synapses," or via signals that remote neurons can interpret. Each one of the neurons has between five and ten thousand synapses. These neurons form networks. Each network has an optimum level of excitement for best function. This level of excitability is controlled by the many hundreds of brain chemicals. Some chemicals increase the excitability of the tissue (i.e., making the tissue more responsive to stimulation), and other chemicals dampen the responsiveness of the tissue. Optimal functioning of any brain tissue relies on a delicate balance between those two opposing effects. Abnormalities in the structure of the brain tissue itself and/or the chemicals bathing them can lead to either increase or decrease in the excitability of one or more of such circuits. The circuit response can thus become too much or too little, relative to the stimulus it receives. In both cases the circuit is behaving abnormally.

It is by now well-recognized that stressors can impair brain function. While the brain is quite capable of handling acute stress (which tends to send the brain into a fight-or-flight mode), it is ill equipped to handle chronic and ongoing stress. It is quite likely that chronic stress (particularly during the early stages of life) changes the balance of inhibition and excitation in one or more neural circuits so that the behavior output dependent on these circuits deviates (Boutros et al, 2015). Until such neural circuits are fully understood, vague psychological notions should be avoided and the urgency of understanding the complex brain circuitry underlying behavior must be stressed. It is much safer to acknowledge ignorance than adopt unsupported notions. As the saying goes, unanswered questions are much less harmful than unquestioned answers.

FORM VS CONTENT

Having practiced psychiatry in two rather different cultural environments and having related to practitioners from every culture, I am struck by the rather high consistency of the forms of psychiatric disorders. A bipolar patient in India, Brazil, Sub-Saharan Africa, or Switzerland will exhibit the same depressive and manic episodes and is likely to respond clinically to the same medications (barring identified genetic variations). This amazing uniformity is what has allowed the development of international nomenclatures like the *DSM (Diagnostic and Statistical Manual)* or the International Classification of Disease (ICD) systems.

This is in marked contrast to the content of delusional material which seems to depend heavily on the cultural background of the individual. While I was practicing in Egypt, manic grandiose delusions were commonly related to having some link to the Prophet Muhammad or one of his major followers or successors. On the other hand, while practicing in the United States, the delusional contents were commonly linked to one of the famous or influential Americans (e.g., The Kennedys or Michael Jackson!).

This suggests that the form of the illness is based on a biology that is common to all humans but the content of the delusions may be derived from the cultural background of the individual. It follows that the neural malfunction needs to be addressed first, and once corrected, then (and perhaps ONLY then) the faulty information content laid down by the faulty neural systems can be corrected through the process of psychotherapy. It is also possible that well-designed psychotherapeutic processes, perhaps over some extended period of time, may be able to correct the aberrant neural systems based on the now well-established brain capacity of plasticity, particularly in younger ages. From this assertion flows another important assertion, and that is to begin therapeutic intervention at the earliest possible opportunity.

The findings and predictions made by Gillberg et al. (1987) are important and worth highlighting at this point. They subjected 20 high functioning children with Autism and Asperger's syndrome to a battery of neurobiological tests as well as a thorough physical examination. Fifteen of the 20 children had "definite abnormalities" on at least one neurobiological test. They concluded that the number of "non-organic" autism cases (i.e., cases where no organic cause can be found based on current day technology), dwindles rapidly as our neurobiological assessment methods become increasingly sophisticated. Research findings over the past several decades indicate that the above statement applies to most known psychiatric disorders.

As a result, it is proposed that the term "NeuroPsychiatric" be adopted to denote all psychiatric conditions resulting from or associated with an identifiable neurological condition. Adopting the term Neuropsychiatry to refer to the entire discipline of Psychiatry, as is recommended by some Neuropsychiatry authorities, would swing the entire field of Psychiatry away from the currently widely adopted BioPsychoSocial model, which looks at socio-environmental factors as well.

Finally, and as indicated by the studies reported in the DSM-IV Source Book, most studies examining disorders with neurological, endocrinological or metabolic interfaces are comprised of small sample sizes. This highlights the fact that major research efforts are yet to be dedicated to further examining the pathophysiology, phenomenology, epidemiology and management of these disorders.

It has been stated that the *DSM* system of diagnosis is 100% reliable (i.e., different clinicians can arrive at the same diagnosis given the same list of symptoms) but 0% valid as none of the categories accurately predicted treatment response or prognosis. Be that as it may, the DSM has allowed clinicians and researchers from all corners of the world to speak a similar language and for patients from all cultures to be included in multicenter-multinational research studies. What is being discussed below regarding "schizophrenia" applies to almost all other psychiatric disorders. Whether terms like OCD and Bipolar disorder survive the revelations from the neurosciences remains to be seen.

SCHIZOPHRENIA: IS IT TIME TO GET RID OF THE TERM?

While the term "Schizophrenia" may have outlasted its usefulness, it is not really time to get rid of it yet. Replacing the term "Schizophrenia" with another term that is equally vague and as inaccurate like "cognitive disorders" "perceptual disorders", or "integration disorders", will not dissipate the stigma or bring us closer to helping those individuals who are suffering from it. On the other hand, there are a number of disorders included under the heading: "schizophrenia." Over the years we have seen smaller and more homogenous (relatively speaking) categories split off this main category. The best example is the split of bipolar disorder (used to be categorized as schizophrenia), followed by the designation of "organic Delusional Disorder and alcoholic hallucinosis) all were once called schizophrenia). Finally, is the split of the Schizoaffective category.

So, as a first step that is already here, clinicians must make sure that accurate diagnoses be made and that non-schizophrenia patients are not labeled that and most crucially not be included in “schizophrenia” study samples. We now can also propose that reasonably well characterized syndromes like the Deficit Syndrome (i.e., schizophrenia patient dominated by what is called negative symptoms like lack of socialization and affect) (Boutros et al. 2014) and drug induced psychosis (Boutros et al. 1996;1998;2009) should also be let out from under the “Schizophrenia” rubric. The term “schizophrenia” should continue to describe the ever-shrinking category of what is believed to be the idiopathic or the genetically inherited syndrome. Eventually we will arrive at a more or less homogenous syndrome with much better understanding of its pathophysiology and if the field would then decide to jettison the term in favor of a more scientific term; I think this would be a most welcome move forward.

The Brain Never Forgets Anything

Chronic Stress Is an Enemy of Healthy Brains: Early Life Stressors Can Result in Enduring Neurophysiological Changes

Early childhood stress has been strongly linked to psychosomatic disorders including conversion disorders like psychogenic non-epileptic seizures (PNES) as well as conditions characterized by dissociation (not remembering what happened during a certain period of time) (Medford, 2014). Early childhood stress, and lifetime assaultive violence have been linked to cortical mal-development and increased electrophysiological abnormalities. Several studies have reported that such severe early stress and abuse to have the potential to alter brain development and cause limbic dysfunction during specific sensitive periods of cortical maturation (Teicher et al. 2003).

The cascade of events is mediated through stress-induced neurohormones of the stress response systems which affects neurogenesis (the growth and development of nervous tissue), synaptic overproduction and myelination (the laying of a cover that enables nerves to transmit information). The aberrant cortical development secondary to stress has been reported to involve a number of brain regions including the corpus callosum connecting the two hemispheres, hippocampus (responsible for memory function), and amygdala (seat of emotions). Over the last decade studies have reported an emergence of EEG abnormalities in children with sexual and psychological abuse (even in the absence of evidence of physical abuse). An increased prevalence of fronto-temporal electrophysiological abnormalities had been reported in abused children, with the abnormalities tending to be localized in the left side of the brain (Teicher et al. 1997). Another study reported EEG abnormalities in 77% of patients who were involved as the child in an incestuous relationship, of which 36% had clinical seizures (Davies 1979). These studies demonstrate the neurobiological mechanisms through which early abuse increases the risk of developing various psychopathologies.

Most recent work strongly supports a relationship between childhood abuse and structural and functional abnormalities in the limbic frontal connectivity resulting in the increased risk for various psychiatric manifestations. Behaviorally, deficient inhibitory control (in a go-nogo paradigm) has also been linked to childhood trauma (Marshall et al. 2016). In the go-nogo experiment the individual is asked to withhold a more natural response (e.g., pushing a button when a particular stimulus appears) in favor of a less natural one (withholding pushing the button when other stimuli, here called non-target, appear). The go-nogo paradigm links cognitive-emotional (i.e., thinking and feeling) networks to the motor output (i.e., doing) of the brain. Utilizing this procedure, Duncan et al. (2015) provided evidence that negative childhood experiences alter prefrontal (cognitive)-insular (emotional)-motor cortical network. While this work was preliminary in scope, it provided tentative bases for the possible link of the aberrant interaction between fronto-limbic cognitive and motoric regions (Duncan et al. 2015) commonly resulting in impulsive and not-well throughout behavior. They proposed that this increased connectivity between fronto-limbic and motor regions could underlie aberrant processing and responsivity to aversive input. Even in the complete absence of evidence, the Biological Principle should still be the driving hypothesis as we proposed regarding conversion or what is otherwise considered hysterical symptoms. As is well-stated by Allen Frances (one of the leading figures of American Psychiatry),"if neuroscience has not yet fully explained psychiatric disorders it is simply because it is yet a bridge too far. Neuroscience will inform everyday Psychiatric diagnosis only at its own slow and steady pace; it cannot be rushed forward before its time-and that time is decidedly not yet". In the meanwhile we cannot fill the gap in our knowledge with unproven and frequently harmful ideas and it is much safer to acknowledge our ignorance not only to ourselves but also to the public.

The Story of the Amnestic Killer

I would like to conclude this chapter with the following amazing case history. Mr. AW was a 32 years old man who was residing in a long-term psychiatric facility for having killed a woman. AW is completely amnestic (i.e., completely unable to remember anything) about the events. During the trial it was revealed that he was under the influence of mind-altering drugs at the time of the crime. AW was in fact a model patient with no abnormal behaviors. He was absolutely cooperative and eventually was trusted to actually work in the vast backyard of the hospital unsupervised. One day, as he was gardening next to one of the roads inside the hospital, a fast car veered off the road and struck him. He was in coma for one week. As he began to awaken, he was noted to be screaming "No, no…." with a sense of real horror. He began to describe re-living the crime that he had never remembered until this moment. He, in fact, gave details of the crime that were never revealed to him. An *EEG* revealed active epileptic activity in the temporal/hippocampal region. The interpretation was that the person's protective brain mechanisms were able to completely suppress the memory that was already weakened by the presence of the mind-altering drugs. The added strength of the epileptic activity emanating from memory-related brain regions seem to have been able to overpower these defense or protective mechanisms allowing the re-emergence of the horrifying details of the crime. The major lesson to be learned is that "it is all there," we just need to learn more about how to access it.

In conclusion, Humanist beliefs allow us to be optimistic regarding the future of the field including accurate prediction, effective prevention, early and accurate diagnosis and treatment. The fact that we are not anywhere close to this vision despite 40 to 50 years of intensive neuroscience research does not by any mean predict that we will never get there. In her book "Mind Fixers: Psychiatry's troubled Search for the Biology of Mental Illnesses", Anne Harrington strongly argues that while there may, indeed, be biological bases for some psychiatric disorders, there must also exist non-biological factors as well. She argues that the intense search for biological bases for any mental disorder is unwise.

I argue that if and when a behavioral deviation is proven not to have a biological basis, it should then not be labeled a psychiatric disorder and treated by biological means (medications or neuromodulatory techniques like electroconvulsive therapy (ECT) or transcranial magnetic stimulation (TMS)). As our neuroevaluative technology is still advancing, declaring a disturbance not to be of a biological nature would be premature, at least for the foreseeable future.

The following anecdote illustrates this. While at Wayne State University I was attending a Neurology Grand Rounds. A prominent neuroradiologist was presenting data on neuroimaging of early Alzheimer patients. He had a cohort of very early Alzheimer patients who were all still fully functioning. He started by showing the computerized axial tomographies (CAT) scans of the patients. They were all perfectly normal! He then showed the magnetic resonance images (MRIs) obtained with the earliest technology of 0.5 tesla (0.5 T) strength. Those also looked rather normal. He followed by showing the MRIs obtained with higher power (1.5 T) and the abnormalities began to become apparent. At this point it still required some expertise in neuroradiology to be able to tell that something was the matter with the scans of those same early and fully functioning patients. At this point he presented the images taken by a 3T powerful MRI system and it no longer required any expertise to see the manifest abnormalities. Upon presenting the MRIs of the same patients, taken at the same time but with a research 4T machine any person, even a lay person, could readily tell that those brains were significantly ill. The field has already advanced and at the time of the writing of this book 7T research MRIs are already being used to explore brain functions.

Chapter 3

WHAT IS IN A NAME?

Prior to the appearance of the DSM system for identifying psychiatric disorders, it was up to each individual clinician to name what they saw happening in an individual patient. Vague terms like *neurosis* and *psychosis* were commonly used. During this era it was not possible for clinicians to share diagnostic impressions without providing many details, which inevitably led a second clinician to reach a different conclusion! As jokingly said; you have ten psychiatrists you get ten different diagnoses! It was also impossible to conduct large scale or multicenter research studies.

THE DSM SYSTEM AND THE MOVE TOWARDS SCIENCE AND BIOLOGY

It has been recognized for decades that medical disorders, particularly neurological and endocrinological disorders, can cause psychiatric symptoms. The history of the development of diagnostic attitudes towards this category of symptoms (i.e., behavioral or cognitive) went through a number of distinct phases. Prior to the Diagnostic and Statistical Manual of Mental Disorders (DSM) era, the fields of psychiatry and Neurology were much closer if not one and the same. Most practitioners were, indeed, neuropsychiatrists. This era is synonymous with such names as Hughlings Jackson, Eugene Bleuler, and Sigmund Freud. This was a time of exploration and discovery. This Neuropsychiatry era was followed by an era that saw an almost complete divorce between Neurology and Psychiatry. In this era, any hint of brain or medical involvement meant that the case was NOT of a psychiatric nature. Most psychiatrists would not care for these patients nor would neurologists. Their care was delegated to other practitioners who were much less qualified and/or interested but who were willing to take care of them. As stated by Denis Hill (Institute of Psychiatry, London) in his introduction to the first edition of *Organic Psychiatry*, "By the turn of the century Psychiatry was overtaken by the immense influence of psychoanalysis" (Lishman, 1987). The most striking example of this era that remains with us today, well into the current medical model era, is care for the mentally retarded. In the USA, mental retardation (now Intellectual Developmental Disability) is not considered part of psychiatry and usually has its own care facilities even separate insurance providers. General psychiatry residents are thus not routinely exposed to issues related to mental retardation. Mental retardation has been neglected in the residency accreditation requirements for adult psychiatry while it was written into the child-psychiatry training requirements in the late 90s (ACGME, 2007). Another stark example of this era that remains with us is the complete delegation of the field of electroencephalography (*EEG*/the recording of the brain's electrical signals) to Neurology despite the well-documented high prevalence of EEG abnormalities in certain psychiatric populations (Shelley et al. 2008).

Since 1952, five Diagnostic and Statistical Manuals of mental disorders have been released by the American Psychiatric Association (APA). Each subsequent edition changed the diagnostic terms and criteria. As can be noticed from the progression described below a serious attempt towards more specificity (i.e., narrower categories) is evident.

Diagnostic and Statistical Manual of Mental Disorders, First Edition (DSM-I)

The DSM-I was published in 1952. Its arrival heralded the move towards evidence-based categorical classification of psychiatric disorders. The basic division in the nomenclature included those mental disorders associated with organic brain disturbance, and those occurring without such primary disturbance of brain function. Further categorization into psychoses, psychoneuroses, and personality disorders was secondary to a more basic division into organic vs. non-organic disorders. As is evident, the dualisms of mind-brain and organic-nonorganic were thus institutionalized in the DSM system.

DSM-I disorders, caused by or associated with impairment of brain tissue function, were all characterized by basic syndromes, consisting of impairment of orientation, impairment of memory, impairment of all intellectual functions (comprehension, calculation, knowledge, learning, etc.), impairment of judgment, or changes in the affect (the outward expression of emotions) where the emotion can either become too shallow relative to the emotion generating it or become too exaggerated and rapidly changing. These syndromes of organic brain disorders are basic mental conditions characteristic of diffuse impairment of brain tissue functions from any cause. They may be mild, moderate, or severe, but most of the basic symptoms of the syndrome are generally present to a similar degree in any one patient at any one time. The severity of the basic syndrome generally parallels the severity of the impairment of brain tissue function.

The organic brain disorders were separated into acute and chronic because of the marked differences between these two groups in regard to prognosis, treatment, and general course of illness. The terms, "acute" and "chronic," refer primarily to the reversibility of brain pathology and its accompanying organic brain syndrome; and not to the cause, onset, or duration of the illness. Since the same cause may produce either temporary or permanent brain damage, a brain disorder which appears reversible, hence acute, at its beginning, may prove later to have left permanent damage and a persistent organic brain syndrome, which will then be diagnosed as chronic.

Diagnostic and Statistical Manual of Mental Disorders, Second Edition (DSM-II)

DSM-II was published by the APA in 1968. The DSM-II readily acknowledged the rapid influx of new knowledge in the field and the evolving nature of any diagnostic system to be developed. The DSM 1l included the concept of Organic Brain Syndromes (OBS), mental disorders caused by or associated with the impairment of brain tissue function. The dichotomy of "organic" vs. "non-organic" was further institutionalized in the second edition of the DSM.

The DSM-II dedicated a section to mental retardation. The classification was based mainly on the severity of the condition with modifiers indicating the possible cause. The *OBS* section was divided into two main categories: psychotic and non-psychotic. The psychotic OBSs included the dementias, alcohol-related disorders, and psychoses associated with neurological conditions like infections, tumors, epilepsy or head injuries. The category also recognized the possibility that endocrinal and metabolic disorders as well as drug use could induce psychotic states. Finally, the OBS category recognized psychosis associated with child birth. The non-psychotic OBSs section recognized the fact that all the causes for psychotic OBSs could also result in non-psychotic OBSs. It should be noted that these categories included OBSs when the condition causing them was not diagnosed. *Schizophrenia* was clearly placed out of the realm of "organically caused" disorders.

Diagnostic criteria included the impairment of orientation, memory, and intellectual functioning, including comprehension, calculation, learning, and knowledge. Judgment was also expected to be impaired as well as the rapid alternation between sadness and elation. *OBSs* were conceived as resulting from "diffuse impairment of brain tissue function from whatever cause."

It is interesting that although the DSM-II recognized an entire category of OBS, a subspecialty of the field to help train physicians to care for these patients did not emerge. Psychiatrists consulting on medical or surgical services were never expected to be the primary treaters of these individuals.

It should be noted that only in 1978 was a textbook dedicated to "Organic Psychiatry" published (Lishman, 1978). In the forward to the first edition, Dennis Hill (Institute of Psychiatry, London), stated, "...across history there have been two main categories of mental disorders, those due to natural or medical causes and those due to supernatural or 'moral' causes."

Diagnostic and Statistical Manual of Mental Disorders, Third Editions (DSM-III and III-R)

The DSM-III, was published in 1980. The dichotomy between "organic" and "mental" continued. In this edition, the DSM went into a multi-axial system where the main diagnosis was on Axis one, permanent or lifelong personality characteristics were on Axis two, any contributing medical condition was on Axis three, psychosocial stressors were listed on Axis four and the level of overall functioning was on Axis five. This was meant to give an overall impression of the level of dysfunction of a patient in one look. For example a *schizophrenia* patient who is doing well and whose disorder is sensitive to environmental stressors would receive the following diagnosis:

Axis one: Schizophrenia.
Axis two: None.
Axis three: None.
Axis four: High stress.

Axis five: 70 (meaning patient remains employed. The lower the number the less functioning is the patient. A patient who receives an overall level of functioning of say 30 is likely to be hospitalized.)

This multi-axial system survived the next two editions to be dispensed with in DSM-5.

Two categories of disorders were relegated to Axis-II. The only common characteristic of the two categories is that they tend to be life-long. Otherwise the two categories of personality disorders and intellectual developmental disorders had no similarities. The major change in the OBS category between DSM II and III was the division of the category into Organic Brain Syndromes (OBSs) and Organic Mental Disorders (OMDs). OBSs refers to a constellation of signs and symptoms without reference to cause (e.g., dementia, delirium), while OMDs is used to refer to OBSs where a cause is known or presumed (e.g., multi-infarct dementia, a loss of cognitive function from damaged blood vessels in the brain.). The essential feature of all these disorders is a "psychological or behavioral abnormality associated with transient or permanent dysfunction of the brain." It is hard to imagine this description not applying to almost all known psychiatric disorders. In the description of the group of disorders, nonetheless, it is stated that "differentiation of OMDs as a separate class does not imply that nonorganic ("functional") mental disorders are somehow independent of brain processes. On the contrary, it is assumed that all psychological processes, normal or abnormal, depend on brain function."

The dilemma our field faces in the continued survival of the mind-brain duality is clearly exemplified. The DSM-III liberalized the concept of organicity and introduced four new diagnostic categories: Organic Affective Syndrome (Organic Mood Disorder in DSM-III-R), Organic Delusional Syndrome, Organic Hallucinosis, and *Organic Personality Syndrome (OPS).* The similarity to "non-organic" disorders was recognized and the need for making the correct diagnosis via accurate evaluations was stressed. Even with the explicit recognition of these disorders, a subspecialty of psychiatry to care for these disorders did not evolve until 1988. The American Neuropsychiatric Association (ANPA), established in 1988, is an organization of professionals in neuropsychiatry, and behavioral neurology. ANPA's mission is to improve the lives of people with disorders at the interface of psychiatry and neurology.

Subsequent to the publication of the DSM-III, the second edition of "Organic psychiatry" was published (Lishman, 1987). In the preface to the second edition, Lishman indicated that "The most remarkable advance since the first edition has come from developments in brain imaging." A plethora of textbooks dedicated to neuropsychiatric disorders soon followed.

A revised edition of the DSM-III (DSM-III-R) was published in 1987. The most interesting observation on the DSM-III-R is the disappearance of the term *Organic Brain Syndrome.* Now the two categories included under "organic" are the Organic Mental Disorders and Organic Mental Syndromes. This is more or less the same classification of the DSM-III. On the other hand, DSM-III-R introduces the hierarchical concept of one disorder or syndrome preempting another (perceived to be of a less pervasive or detrimental nature). Based on the hierarchical model, the presence of an organic (i.e., based on a brain dysfunction) disorder trumps the "functional or not based on a brain disorder" disorder it resembles. This stipulation has far reaching diagnostic and possibly legal ramifications as the failure of a physician to perform the proper "organic" workup and missing the "organic" diagnosis would not be defensible based on the DSM-III-R.

DSM-III-R continues nonetheless to exhibit the difficulty facing our field as long as the field continues to subscribe to the mind-brain duality. While the so called "organic" disorders are clearly attributable to brain dysfunctions, "functional" disorders can be results of behavioral, psychological or biological factors. The DSM-III-R immediately follows the last assertion with another assertion that it believes all psychological, and behavioral facets are based on brain functions. This straddling the fence attitude leaves the door wide open for the mind-brain duality to continue to prosper. In the intervening years between the printing of the

DSM-III-R and the DSM-IV the American Neuropsychiatric Association saw a significant rise in its membership with many practicing psychiatrists recognizing that care for these patients on the fence between psychiatry and neurology is not only profitable and helpful to the patient, but also that this area of psychiatry can no longer be ignored by the average psychiatrist.

DIAGNOSTIC AND STATISTICAL MANUAL OF MENTAL DISORDERS, FOURTH EDITIONS (DSM-IV AND ITS TEXT REVISION DSM-IV-TR)

In 1994, the APA published the fourth edition of the *DSM* (DSM-IV). The major change introduced in the DSM-IV is the disappearance of the term "Organic." The "organic' category was replaced by three categories: the first group of cognitive disorders like delirium, dementia, and amnesia; and the second category is that of "Mental Disorders Due to a General Medical Condition (GMC)." The third category is that of substance-related disorders. There was absolutely no recognition of any biological processes leading to a substance abuse disorder. Addiction was not seen as an organic brain problem but instead a problem caused solely by the use of drugs.

The struggle with the mind-brain dichotomy continues in the DSM-IV nonetheless as the continued use of the term "mental" indicates. As with the DSM-III and III-R the DSM-IV includes in Appendix-A a number of decision trees for differential diagnoses. Common among the trees is an essential requirement, as a mandatory first step, to make sure that the presenting symptoms are not "due to the direct physiological effects of a general medical condition or GMC." Nowhere in the manual is the level of the evidence linking the GMC and the psychiatric manifestations outlined.

Moreover, the requirement that the GMC fully explains the symptoms contradicts the bio-psychosocial conceptualization of psychiatric disorders, which recognizes the complex interactions between social and psychological factors on one end and the biology of the brain on the other. The only exception made in DSM-IV to this rule is for substance-induced disorders where it is recognized that both psychiatric and GMC can contribute to complications of substance use. These categories did not significantly change in the revised text edition of the DSM-IV (DSM-IV-TR) published in 2000. It is of interest to note that the DSM-IV Organic Mental Disorders work group was renamed the "Cognitive Impairment Disorders" work group. This new name is equally unfortunate as it does not recognize the fact that brain changes can affect emotions and behavior even in the absence of cognitive changes.

DSM-5

The struggle with the mind-brain dichotomy continues in the DSM-5 nonetheless as the continued use of the term "mental" indicates, but with an interesting caveat. The designation that a "condition" is due to a General Medical Condition was modified to the "condition" being secondary to "another" medical condition. The term "General" is removed and term "another" is used; implicitly recognizing that the "mental" condition is in fact a "medical" condition. The group of disorders comprised of delirium, dementia, and amnestic as well as other cognitive disorders are now categorized under a new section "Neurocognitive disorders," with a new subcategory for "mild" impairments. The third group which is substance use disorder continues without the slightest recognition of the biological bases of addictive behavior.

Conclusion and Implications for the *DSM-6* and Beyond

The mind-brain dichotomy continues to plague our conceptualization of psychiatric disorders. The *DSM-IV Source Book* (a rather large volume listing all the references used to arrive at the various categories) stated that "as of the development of this version the organic nature of many psychiatric disorders has not been demonstrated" (APA, 1994). The firm recognition of neuropsychiatric disorders as "psychiatric" and that caring for these individuals is well within the scope of professional skills a psychiatrist should have, definitely resolves the mind-brain issue for the field of Neuropsychiatry. Neuropsychiatry as a subspecialty of psychiatry focused on diagnosing and managing patients on the borderline between psychiatry and neurology indeed remains in its infancy. It should be highlighted that disorders that appear neuropsychiatric prior to evaluation (example, conversion symptoms), are not labeled "neuropsychiatric" once the work up proves completely negative for a neurological cause of the symptoms. The most recent development of a subspecialty certification in Neuropsychiatry and Behavioral Neurology is a most hopeful step in the right direction.

Terminology like "neuropsychiatry" yields itself to describing a number of conditions where, for example, an endocrine (e.g., thyroid disorder), or metabolic (e.g., porphyria, a disorder that can cause nerve or skin problems) factor contributes to the disorder by using modified terms like Psychoendocrine or Psychometabolic disorder, leaving the term "Psychiatric" to describe all other disorders where a specific cause has not yet been identified.

Chapter 4

A Humanist Model for the Practice of Psychiatry: A Proposal to Facilitate Assimilation of New Knowledge

Generalists and Specialization

Psychiatry as a clinical discipline is ever expanding with many sub areas gaining huge bodies of scientific knowledge. The number of specialized peer-reviewed journals addressing a particular area of psychiatry is multiplying with 4-6 journals each specializing in mood, psychosis, anxiety, personality, neuropsychiatry, addiction, children and adolescents, eating, and sexual disorders with on-line-only (i.e., open access) journals continuously being added. It is thus not possible for any one clinician to stay abreast of all that gets published in this ever-increasing number of journals (currently about 250). In addition, scientific organizations with particular emphasis on one or the other of these areas are constantly sprouting. The basic assumption (a widely held one in the current environment) that such journals and societies are mainly "research" oriented and not very useful for the average practicing clinician is, in fact, false. Many of these organizations strive to be clinically relevant. In fact, a psychiatrist who happens to see a particular type of patients would benefit a great deal of reading such journals and belonging to the organization pertinent to his/her area of interest.

It follows that due to the rapidly expanding bulk of knowledge, specialized psychiatrists are necessary. The generalists remain a very important part of the system, as they become the main contact point for the patient's first interaction with the system. However, the generalists need to know the limitations of their knowledge and must be able to consult with or refer patients to more specialized professionals when necessary.

This is particularly essential for medical school settings. While a small number of highly regarded medical schools have specialized divisions (more than just adult and child or inpatient and outpatient) the overwhelming number of medical schools don't. I here propose the following to be the standard for any medical school entrusted with teaching future generations of physicians. An academic department of psychiatry must, at a minimum, have specialists in psychotic disorders, mood disorders, anxiety disorders, personality disorders, and addiction disorders. That still leaves many subspecialty areas of psychiatry uncovered. The fields of eating disorders, psychosexual disorders, forensic psychiatry, and neuropsychiatry are also very important and whenever possible should be included in medical school teaching as well. The above applies equally to the various areas of child and adolescent psychiatry.

The Relation to Medicine, Particularly Neurology and Endocrinology

The fields of neurology and endocrinology are particularly closely related to psychiatry. Neuroendocrinology is currently severely underemphasized in psychiatric training. There are no specific knowledge areas that are mandated to be included in the resident education curricula, despite the well-known relationship between the cortico-adrenal axis and anxiety/depression on the one hand and thyroid and pituitary-related psychiatric manifestations on the other. To my knowledge, there are no psychoneuroendocrinology fellowship programs currently in the United States and neuroendocrinology fellowships are not open for psychiatrists, despite the presence of an international organization for psychoneuroendocrinology and a number of scientific journals catering to this area of knowledge.

Luckily, this is not the case for neuropsychiatry. There is a sub-specialization Board "The American Board of Behavioral Neurology and NeuroPsychiatry" administered by the American Board of Neurological Subspecialties. In contrast to psychoneuroendocrinology, a number of scientific journals and at least two international organizations are dedicated to this sub-specialty.

Should Psychiatry and Neurology Be Re-Integrated?

While there is no doubt that psychiatry, neurology, and neurosurgery are clinical neuroscience disciplines, psychiatry by any measure is a rather unique field. After finishing my psychiatry residency, neurology residency and behavioral neurology and clinical neurophysiology fellowships, I finally had to choose a main department to belong to and a secondary department to affiliate with. The decision was extremely difficult. Two factors made belonging to neurology appealing; better pay and better status (higher respect) within the medical community. In 1985, the year I had to decide, both the American Academy of Neurology (AAN) and the American Psychiatric Association (APA) Annual Meetings were coming to Dallas, where I happened to be working. The

AAN occupied the largest hotel downtown but the APA occupied the entire downtown.

The APA was an impressive event with 15,000 psychiatrists, continuous and simultaneous presentations from 7AM to 9 PM for 6 days. The absolutely dizzying breadth of the field was immediately apparent; from presentations tackling the most sophisticated neuroscience techniques and advances to the most psychodynamic and cross-cultural political sciences. The decision was clear. Psychiatry was such a large and broad field that room for research (my interest) was vast. It also has become clear that the field is too large and the bulk of knowledge pertinent to everyday clinical work is simply too large to be mastered by individual clinicians. In other words, sub-specialization in psychiatry is inevitable and is the way for the future. It is thus hard to imagine this expanding already vast field joining another similarly expanding and vast disciplines (i.e., Neurology).

What, in fact, has already happened is that the field of neuropsychiatry has been born. This subspecialty of psychiatry has its sister in the neurology discipline of behavioral neurology. Each of the two disciplines has its own organizations and specialty journals. The wonderful news is that the two organizations are friendly and do meet jointly occasionally. Moreover, the two organizations have recently collaborated in developing a subspecialty board certification in behavioral neurology/neuropsychiatry open for both neurologists and psychiatrists. Hence, I think the two disciplines of psychiatry and neurology have already found their way to collaborating where enough common ground exists.

Having consistently had joint psychiatry/neurology faculty appointments, I had the experience of bright psychiatry residents being lured away, particularly to neurology with the invitation to jump ship "You are so good. What are you doing in psychiatry?"

Future Psychiatry is an intense neuroscience-based discipline. The NIMH has declared that psychiatric disorders are neuro-circuitry disorders. Hence, it will not be too far in the future when a competent psychiatrist will need to be able to identify the neural dysfunction(s) of a particular patient. In order to accomplish that, a clinician will need to have thorough knowledge of neuroanatomy, neurophysiology, neurochemistry and neuropharmacology. He/she will also need to be able to utilize the available diagnostic technology masterfully, from genetic testing to fMRI (functional Magnetic Resonance Imaging), PET (positron emission tomography) scanning, magnetic resonance spectroscopy (MRS), EEG and magnetoencephalography (MEG). I would not be surprised if, at some time in the future, psychiatry residencies become a five-year intensive program. Psychiatry residency programs are currently four years and do not include teaching of any of the aforementioned techniques.

EMBRACING TECHNOLOGY

There is little doubt that the ever-advancing brain imaging and genetic testing technologies will revolutionize the practice of clinical psychiatry. We witnessed the progression of brain imaging from the CT-scans to the MRI.5 tesla to the current three-tesla scanners in common use. Four-tesla scanners are already here, and studies utilizing higher magnetic power of up to seven-tesla power is already appearing. With each advance in the magnetic power, amazing details are revealed in the scanned brains.

Magnetic resonance spectroscopy (MRS) carries the promise of examining the neurochemistry of individual patients and makes the possibility of personalized prescribing just over the horizon. Functional magnetic resonance imaging (fMRI) promises the ability to test every neuroanatomical structure to very precisely identify the dysfunctional brain regions in a particular individual. This is particularly exciting in the era of brain stimulation.

The rapidly advancing brain stimulation technology promises the ability to manipulate (for therapeutic reasons) a particular brain region or circuit that is thought to be dysfunctional. Such technology now ranges from least invasive like direct current transcranial brain stimulation (tDCS) and transcranial magnetic stimulation (TMS) to more invasive technologies like vagal nerve stimulation (VNS) and deep brain stimulation (DBS).

Electroconvulsive therapy (ECT) has been a stable of psychiatric treatment for decades. The side effects are well documented, which prevent many patients who could benefit from ECT from getting the treatment. The advancing technology of magnetic seizure therapy (MST) promises to ameliorate the side effects while maintaining the therapeutic benefits. It is crucial that current day practicing psychiatrists be aware of these advances and help their institutions adopt them as they accrue the necessary evidence for safety and efficacy.

What is being proposed here is much easier to be adopted in academic institutions prior to spreading to private practice settings. But change is always difficult. In my opinion the current governing structure of academic institutions is an obstacle to change as is described below.

Governance of Academic Departments of Psychiatry

When I began to interact with the academic healthcare system in the USA almost 50 years ago, soon after arriving from my homeland, Egypt, I was struck by the fact that academic medical departments, and perhaps all academic university departments, are more or less forms of dictatorship without a major democratic process. In my many positions in a number of psychiatry departments I found myself in conflict with the chairperson of the department. Given that there were no processes to discuss grievances or conflicts, the conflicts and problems tended to fester. This usually led the faculty member to leave for a different university which was usually willing to offer incentives to gain an already trained faculty member. The relocation of a faculty member, particularly a productive and successful one, is a significant loss to both the institution that had actually invested its resources in developing the faculty member's career and also a loss to the faculty member him/herself as he/she had to leave behind many acquaintances, collaborators, and trained personnel.

Humanist ideology highly values the democratic process. It would make sense that the governance of academic departments be a democratic process. A number of methodologies can be developed to assure that. For instance, a committee of tenured and non-tenured (if this category exists in a particular academic institution) professors could be formed to be advisors to the chairperson in all matters related to governing the department. Conflicts would thus not be seen as conflicts with one person but with an entire committee. This would be much harder to be seen as personal and thus result less in the departure of productive and valued faculty members.

The current ladder system of promotions in academic departments is also problematic. The current system calls for a three-step system in most institutions. Usually, a person is initially hired at the assistant professor level and then promoted to associate professor and the final step is full professor. Many departments thus end up with many professors and tend to become "top-heavy." A number of institutions have remedied this problem by adding additional steps. For example, having different professorial levels like professor step one or professor step two and so on. I'm proposing that all academic faculty be hired initially at the assistant instructor level then promoted to instructor then to assistant professor-I followed by assistant professor-II prior to being promoted to associate professor-I. Associate professor-II would precede the promotion to full professor. Full professors would then be candidates for promotion to chair-professors. Governance of an academic department could then be the job of a committee of the chair-professors with a rotating overall chair of the committee. In this system, no department would actually recruit a chairperson but only recruit at the ranks leading up to chair-personhood.

The future of Psychiatry is expensive and the dilemma of evidence-base: whose responsibility, is it?

As was mentioned before the National Institutes of Mental Health (NIMH) has defined psychiatric disorders as neurocircuitry disturbances. Functional imaging technology is rapidly characterizing and defining the millions of neural circuits sub-serving the many higher cortical functions. As the NIMH definition invokes these circuits, it is fully expected that the deviations in specific circuits, underlying certain cognitive or emotional deviations in the more common or what are now named serious mental illnesses, will eventually be characterized. Evidence is also growing that similar advances are being made for childhood disorders (Balsters et al. 2016).

Hence, it follows that when a particular individual begins to exhibit a certain behavioral deviation, functional neuroimaging should be employed to identify the disturbed neural circuits. Furthermore, such rapidly advancing technologies are very likely to be able to point out individuals at high risk for developing psychiatric disorders, thus allowing the medical profession to intervene at a very early stage of disease development. The fMRI technology has also demonstrated an ability to probe such disorders as pedophilia raising the hope that such individuals (who tend to languish in institutions) may be diagnosable and treatable (Poeppl et al. 2012). Furthermore, such imaging techniques are highly likely to be capable eventually of predicting relapse and thus be very useful in maintaining the recovery of individual patients.

The rapidly advancing brain neuromodulation methodology will eventually allow targeting a circuit or groups of circuits. In fact, such neuromodulatory technologies already have been hybridized with other diagnostic modalities for even greater accuracy and reliability of mapping the various brain functions. It also follows that once the circuitry disturbances have been diagnosed prior to treatment, such tests will need to be repeated following treatment to assess the efficacy. Imagine the cost of care for a single patient who is in need of deep brain stimulation (DBS) for treatment refractory depression or obsessive-compulsive disorder (OCD). Starting with an intense and exhaustive clinical review with more than one qualified clinician agreeing on the need for DBS, the case will need to be reviewed by an ethics committee before the go ahead for the work-up and procedure can commence. Then there are imaging procedures, neurosurgery, and consultation leading to the actual procedure. A close follow up will also be necessary. Even less expensive (and much less invasive) procedures like transcranial magnetic stimulation (TMS) could prove quite expensive as patients usually need daily treatments for weeks (4-6 weeks) before a solid response is attained.

In other words, early diagnosing and instituting effective treatment, as well as relapse prediction and prevention will all heavily depend on expensive treatment (hopefully less expensive in the future than the current cost due to more widespread use and decreases in the cost of the equipment), but will all add up to a more scientifically based, more effective field, albeit one that is more expensive than any other field of medicine.

Evidence Bases Can Be a Double-Edged Sword

How will such costly diagnostic and therapeutic procedures filter down from the research world to the clinical world? Not too long ago, the standard for adopting a procedure was almost entirely based on the clinicians' experiences. Obviously, that is a flawed system that has led to many procedures being adopted prematurely. Over time, evidence-based practices replaced the physicians' judgments. This also is not devoid of problems. How much evidence is needed for a procedure to be adopted? Does cost or invasiveness affect the decision or is it largely based on benefit for the patient?

Evidence has been categorized into levels. Anecdotal reports are considered the lowest and least reliable evidence. Larger and more systematized case studies carry slightly higher evidentiary value. Controlled studies also have different levels progressively higher values from open-label, single-blind to double blind randomized controlled studies (DB-RCT). DB-RCTs are extremely expensive to perform. More expensive still are multi-center DB-RCTs. Hence, the major question is whose responsibility is it to fund such studies and what sort of evidence is necessary for the responsible agency to be morally obligated to fund such studies? This point strongly highlights the need that all medical schools be qualified and incentivized to participate in such studies.

As is well-known, the current funding environment is extremely challenging. Let's consider a scenario where a number of anecdotal reports have appeared that drug A is beneficial in condition X. Conducting an open label study at this point should not be very expensive but is highly unlikely to be funded by the NIH or by pharmaceutical companies (as drug A is already generic). Currently, the agency and the field rely on the goodness of a few clinical academic departments that are willing to shoulder the cost. At this stage, and assuming the open label study is supportive of the efficacy of drug A, replication studies are still needed. A rare private foundation may also come to the rescue of disorder X, facilitating the more labor intensive and expensive controlled studies. There are no guidelines of how many open label replications are needed before more expensive, controlled/blinded studies become necessary, and then how many of these are sufficient for a procedure or treatment to be adopted?

Chapter 5

A Proposed New System of Integrated Psychiatric Care with Prevention, Primary Care, General Psychiatry Practice, Specialization and Sub-Specialization: From Pre-Conception to Terminal Care

The proposed Integrated Psychiatric Care System has four levels: primary prevention, primary care, general psychiatric care, and sub-specialized to super-specialized psychiatric care. Two essential elements are necessary for adequate psychiatric care for everyone; de-stigmatization and prevention. De-stigmatization as well as prevention require a global and universal mental health-psychiatric care plan.

PRIMARY PREVENTION

Based on the concepts that all children's welfare is the responsibility of the state delegated to the family, and that the majority of (if not all) psychiatric disorders have their roots in childhood, the following proposal is developed. This system is based on the development of a cadre of well-qualified family counselors/social workers. Every family who is planning to have a child or is in the process of having a child is assigned a counselor. The counselor's job is to advise regarding pre-natal care and assure that the family has the resources necessary for proper nutrition for mother and child. This is a crucial stage and an important element of the proposal. Use of alcohol during pregnancy can result in the fetal alcohol syndrome (FAS). The prevalence of FAS in the general population is estimated to be 7.7 per 1000 individuals and was reported to be highest among Europeans with an estimate of 19.8/1000 (Lange et al. 2017). It is a lifelong disability that is completely preventable. Similar issues are related to opioid use during pregnancy. How effective the presence of the counselor is will need to be borne out by longitudinally well-designed follow-up studies.

Once the child is born healthy, the job of the counselor is to act as a resource for the family in case of need. Routine pediatric visits and immunizations can be tracked via computer systems. Computers should flag a child who is delinquent on immunizations or fails to have the required pediatric routine checkups. The role of the counselor remains restricted to an annual wellness visit to the family. If there are no indications of problems, then routine visits continue. If there are indications of problems, then the counselor's job is to marshal resources to assist the family. The purpose is to assure the health and well-being of the children.

Once there are no longer children in the picture (i.e., all children are 18 and above), counselors no longer do house visits but remain available for a once-a-year session with the parents. The focus now should be on the continued welfare of the marriage and if there are any early warning signs of any psychiatric issues. With mutual agreement, such visits can become optional. A counselor will always be assigned and available for the family.

When a psychiatric condition is identified (or suspected), the counselor becomes a case manager in coordinating the care of the patient, care givers, and significant others. Again, a major role for the counselor is to make sure all resources available are marshaled to bear on the problem at hand. A counselor will thus be always assigned to the family into older adulthood and be involved in end of life care.

COUNSELORS

It is obvious that different sets of skills will be needed by counselors serving at different stages. Families are handed from one stage counselors to the next throughout life.

The Early-Stage Counselor

Counselors at this stage should be trained on detecting signs of problems, particularly all forms of abuse. Counselors' major task is assuring that the children are getting all necessary care. As counselors are not expected to function as health professionals, their role is limited to identify problems and help families obtain proper care. It is of great importance that the family views the counselor as a helpful resource and does not develop a paranoid attitude towards him/her. This obviously requires significant training on many aspects including cultural sensitivity.

Counselors of Post Childhood Stages

Counselors at this stage are dealing mainly with adults. The main function here is the primary prevention of psychiatric disorders by identifying life situations that are likely to lead to the development of such problems and ameliorating them if possible. Again, the counselors are NOT medical professionals so their main function is identifying ongoing stressors and helping to marshal resources for the alleviation of stress. The second major function is both the early identification of psychiatric disorders and early intervention when warning signs are detected. A level of awareness of early symptoms would be necessary for counselors working at this stage.

Counselors at the Older Adult and End of Life Stages

The main skill common to all stages is the full awareness of community resources available to help the family cope with stressors. Counselors at this stage would also extend their care to individuals in senior citizens housing, assisted living, and skilled nursing facilities.

PRIMARY CARE

As is already well known most psychiatric care is provided by general practitioners and family physicians. This is in agreement with Humanistic concepts as well as good medical practice. The system proposed above should bring an individual with early warning signs of a disorder to medical care. Data will need to be developed as to when a patient should be moved from a primary care to a general psychiatry setting.

GENERAL PSYCHIATRY

Psychiatrists can be generalists or specialists. All individuals with psychiatric illnesses who are in need of care, should be evaluated by a general psychiatrist (heretofore called GPsy). The major bulk of psychiatric care should be provided by GPsy. It is essential that criteria be developed for when the care of a patient must move from GPsy to sub- or super specialization level. It should be fully understood that continuing care would always be provided by GPsy once the special sub or super specialty expertise is no longer needed.

SUB AND SUPER-SPECIALIZED PSYCHIATRIC CARE

Sub-specialized psychiatrists provide the next level upward in care of complex and difficult patients. A patient may be seen by a psychiatrist with advanced training in thought, mood, anxiety, personality, addiction, or neuropsychiatric disorders. These specialists must function as general community resources with local and state-wide consultation facilitated.

A final category of select psychiatrists with super-specialization (mainly in major academic centers), should also be available to bear on the care of the most difficult and treatment-resistant patients. A thought disorder specialist may develop additional expertise, for example, in delusional or schizoaffective disorders. Similarly, an anxiety disorder specialist may develop additional expertise in Panic Disorder, PTSD or OCD. Super-specialized psychiatrists should function as general resources for the field with statewide or nationwide consultation possible. Figure one below illustrates the proposed flow of care from the least to the most specialized thus affording the most sophisticated care to the most difficult patients.

Humanistic psychiatric care is undoubtedly expensive but the alleviation of human suffering is to be viewed as paramount. Consonant with the scientific requirements for Humanistic care, complete data must be kept and statistics must be examined to provide evidence that the system is making a difference in alleviating suffering.

Here I would like to discuss the issue this program will surely raise: the big brother issue, the fear of intrusion into privacy as well as of the intrusion of government into our private lives. There is no doubt that any system, no matter how benevolent, can be abused. This is not enough reason, by itself, to keep from developing new and possibly useful programs. Safeguards must be put in place to avoid the system being used for unacceptable purposes. On the other hand, the system is humanistically mandated as the well-being of children supersedes privacy concerns by adults. Leaving children's welfare up to the parents is a rejected concept. Delegating care responsibility to the parents is acceptable as long as a system is in place to detect when such a responsibility is not being discharged. Cases in point are when parents deny children medical care based on religious beliefs. Courts have always sided with the scientific knowledge that proper medical care be made available. These cases clearly demonstrate that in fact, the laws do see the state as the ward of the children and not their parents.

Notes on the Vital Role of State Psychiatric Hospitals

The main concern with the majority of state hospitals is the de-emphasized role of research and teaching as well as the general inability to recruit top notch clinicians. This is particularly important as the most severely ill patients end up in these facilities generating a pernicious sense of hopelessness among both patients and care providers. While research and academic affiliations' beneficial roles are usually mentioned in many of the mission statements, that is hardly the emphasis or practice. In my opinion much more is necessary.

State Hospitals Serve Unique Populations

Only a small minority of psychiatric patients ever receive care from state facilities. Patients at a state hospital are characterized by their level of complexity and/or legal involvement. Hence, these factors make this particular population not highly suitable for "Hypotheses Driven Research," the sort of research likely to get funded by national or federal agencies. This means slower progress, if any, in understanding the complex nature of the patients being treated and developing more effective therapies geared specifically towards these populations. As the field of Psychiatry is ever advancing state hospital patients should be among the first to benefit from advances in the field and not the absolute last. Special emphasis must be placed on trying to understand the complex Bio-Psycho-Social interplay including developing methodologies to confidently differentiate between non-psychiatric and psychiatric criminal behavior (psychopathy is included under psychiatric).

A much higher emphasis needs to be placed on rehabilitation, informed and guided by the latest research findings. State hospitals should be in the forefront of cognitive and work rehabilitation. Much needed data can be generated in the course of administering and monitoring the various forms of rehabilitation.

Finally, research needs to be conducted on the effects of the living environment on outcome. While much gets said regarding treatment in the "least restrictive environment" the majority of state hospitals house patients in ward-like environments with a relatively small number of much wider living spaces, like cottages.

A number of factors have led to the paucity of research in state facilities: recruiting non-academically oriented clinicians, a lack of research support, and additional research requirements over and above what the affiliated university requires. It should be noted that the majority of state hospitals have no academic affiliations.

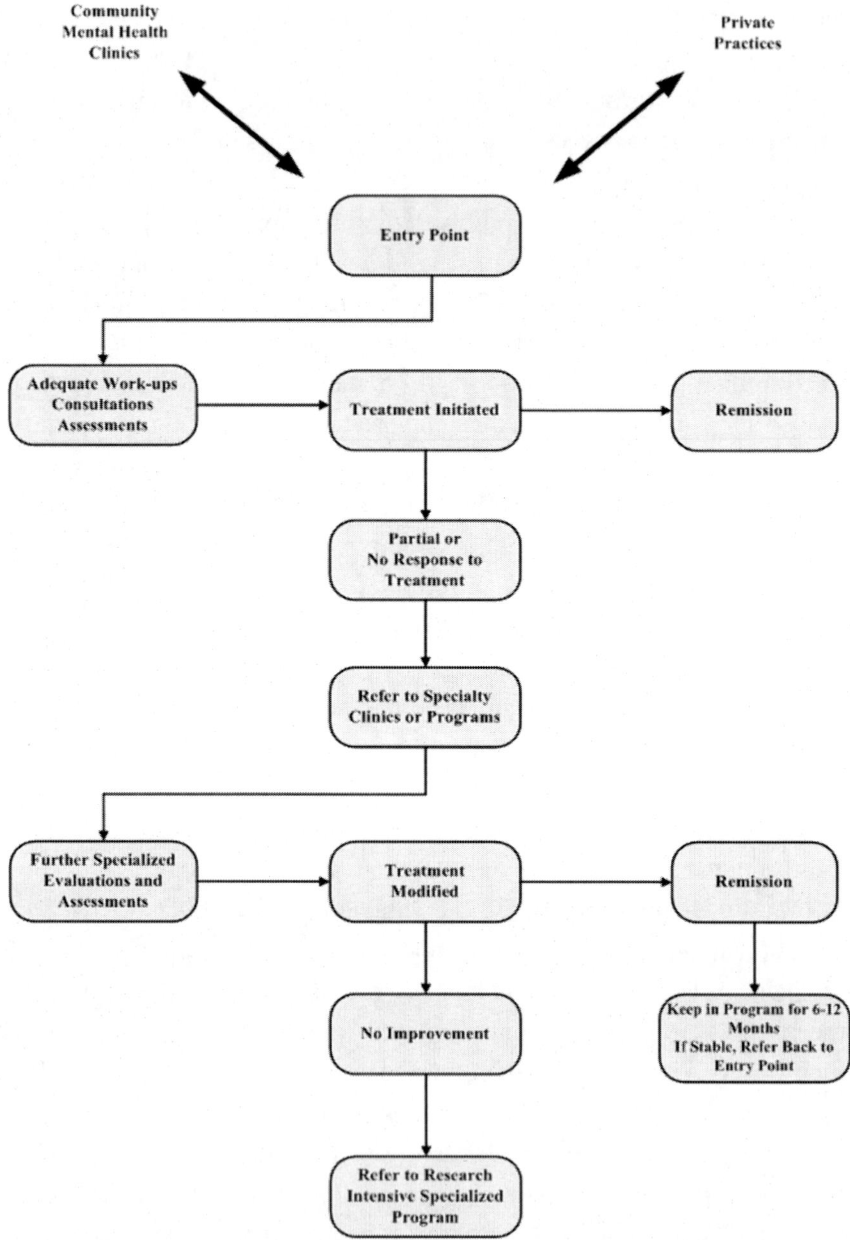

Figure 1. Illustrates the proposed flow of care from the least to the most specialized thus affording the most sophisticated care to the most difficult patients.

Problem of the Inverted Pyramid

Due to financial reasons and due to work environments, most brilliant clinicians either end up in private practice or in intensive research institutions. This leaves us with an inverted pyramid where the least sick get the best care while the sickest tend to end up in state facilities.

Different state hospitals or different states may have different populations or unique problems. Hence, research in these facilities must be driven locally by the special needs of each facility and with oversight provided by public-academic collaboration.

The adoption of new diagnostic and therapeutic technology needs to be facilitated. For example, with so much organic brain involvement in state hospital populations, computer-based neuropsychological assessments and computer-based cognitive rehabilitations has become within reach.

RECOMMENDATIONS

1. There is a need for a much more serious emphasis on the academic-public collaboration. The mere affiliation with a medical school, while very likely to improve the caliber of clinicians providing the clinical care, does not necessarily assure that an environment of LEARNING AND INQUISITVENESS will be created. Such an environment could have many beneficial effects besides the research being conducted. A stimulating environment will affect all mental health workers in the environment.
2. Scholarly activity can and perhaps should involve all disciplines and NOT be limited to physicians and psychologists.
3. Significant funding specifically earmarked to support clinical research in state facilities is likely to result in attracting bright and committed physicians and psychologists. This funding would

be used to support research initiatives that address one of the unique populations served by the system and can potentially lead to furthering the understanding of the pathology or developing more effective treatment modalities.

4. Specialized fellowship programs should be developed to help generate a cadre of clinicians thoroughly familiar with state facilities' populations, regulations, and resources. A state hospital fellowship program would include rotations on medium and long-term units, forensic services, special exposure to issues related to sexual offenders, fully evaluating and developing treatment and rehab programs for individuals with significant brain damage (developmental or acquired), administrative issues and state facilities research regulations.
5. A specific mechanism to adopt new treatment modalities (whether psychological or somatic) would assure both proper and early implementation, and generate data regarding the efficacy of the treatment in this particular setting. Many concepts have face value appeal but must be subjected to rigorous evaluations before being accepted as "effective." Once a treatment modality is accepted as effective in well-controlled studies or specific populations, work must then proceed to define the implementation strategies, stages of implementation, and ways to monitor the effectiveness of the implemented program. It is essential that individuals implementing a program (whether a new medication or, for example, trauma-informed therapy) be fully aware of the evidence that supports their work. This assures a level of confidence and commitment that is likely to be transmitted not only to the patients but also their families and care-givers.
6. All state hospitals must have the ability to graduate patients from restrictive ward environment to more community-like living spaces. The impact of being able to do so needs to be examined and documented.

7. As part of being one with the community of care, state hospitals can also become sources for education to the healing communities where they exist.

CONCLUSION

State hospital patients present unique populations that are seriously under served in terms of research. Providing more funds to state facilities must be accompanied by a qualitative change in philosophy, creating an environment of learning and inquisitiveness. State hospitals must not be places to warehouse difficult and unresponsive patients BUT must be places for learning and teaching that create excitement and hope for a better future. While state hospitals remain sorely needed, progress towards their eventual elimination will not happen unless the unique issues of these facilities and the system as a whole are probed in a careful and systematic manner.

Chapter 6

SHOULD PSYCHIATRY BE A SEPARATE SCHOOL FROM MEDICINE?

Currently, psychiatry is a branch of Medicine. In order to be a psychiatrist a physician must first complete medical school then join a residency program. Residency programs are usually four years in duration. Additional specialization, as in child psychiatry or in geriatric psychiatry requires an additional year for clinical competence or two years if research competence is to be gained as well. A total duration of training of approximately 12 years is thus required to become a general psychiatrist.

NATURE OF PSYCHIATRY

Psychiatry as a field differs fundamentally from other branches of medicine. While medical fields like internal medicine, surgery, or pediatrics all require thorough knowledge of the anatomy, physiology, and the biochemistry of all organ systems of the human body, the current day practice of psychiatry does not require such thorough knowledge of organs like the stomach or liver.

Schools of psychiatry would be four-year schools following college. A student who has completed a pre-medical requirement could apply to this school. The curriculum should cover a wide range of topics allowing the student to develop a wide range of knowledge covering all of the possible basic sciences required to be able to understand psychiatric disorders and conduct meaningful research to advance the field.

AREAS TO BE COVERED

Basic neurobiology of the brain including anatomy, physiology and neurochemistry. Neuropharmacology should be covered in detail. Psychology should also be covered in detail. The first two years of the school of psychiatry should be devoted to the basic sciences. The last two years of the school should be devoted to clinical sciences.

The graduates will need to go for a one year internship. At this point, they are ready to practice general clinical psychiatry. Most graduating individuals should be encouraged to go for an additional two years of advanced training in a specialty area.

The above proposed setup will lead to the generation of two classes of practicing psychiatrists. The first class would be comprised of general psychiatrists. General psychiatrists would function as the main gatekeepers of the field. All patients will need to be initially evaluated by a general psychiatrist. Simple and readily responsive cases could be managed by a general psychiatrist or referred back to the general practitioner while more difficult cases and treatment resistant ones could then be referred to a specialist. A general psychiatrist should be reasonably well-versed in all aspects of the field of psychiatry and should be able to recognize difficult on complex cases early upon presentation.

Psychiatry subspecialties would include the following (and these would constitute departments in the School of Psychiatry with chairs and faculty).

1. Child psychiatry.
2. Consultation liaison psychiatry.
3. Forensic psychiatry.
4. Thought disorders.
5. Affective disorders.
6. Anxiety disorders.
7. Personality disorders.
8. Addiction and substance use disorders.
9. Psychosexual disorders.
10. Neuropsychiatric disorders.
11. Psychiatric electrophysiology.
12. Psychiatric neuroimaging.
13. Neuro endocrine and neurometabolic disorders including eating disorders.

It is immediately obvious that each one of these areas is a vast area of knowledge that is rapidly expanding. It is thus expected that further sub specialization within each one of these areas would eventually become necessary. For example, within the field of neuropsychiatric disorders it can be easily envisioned that one physician may specialize in treating head injured individuals while another would focus on psychiatric patients with epilepsy or stroke.

A fundamental difference between the two groups of psychiatrists would be that the generalists continue to be clinical practitioners and serve mainly in the community, while the specialists would serve tertiary and quaternary medical centers as well as medical schools.

An additional model that could be considered would be to form three-categories. The three-category system would, in addition to the generalists and the specialists, generate a category of academic psychiatrists. The main distinguishing elements of an academic psychiatrist would be the combination of the clinical and the academic degrees. Thus, an academic psychiatrist would have a Ph.D. degree in addition to the clinical degree. This would be a requirement to hold an academic position in a teaching/research institution. To a large extent most of these institutions tend to be supported by taxpayer money and acquiring academically trained and qualified faculty would assure the productivity of such faculty.

The two-tier system implies that all specialists would be academically trained and would be required to participate in advancing and disseminating knowledge about psychiatric disorders.

The above proposal could help ease the current shortage of psychiatrists nationwide. Not only that it is a faster and less costly system, it more than likely will be able to generate highly qualified practitioners.

Chapter 7

Psychiatric Education

The National Institute of Mental Health (NIMH) repeatedly indicated a difficulty in recruiting psychiatrists into research. The NIMH cites three main factors for this problem: financial issues, lack of mentorship, and the failure of current teaching curricula in connecting clinical psychiatry with relevant science.

The problem is more pervasive. I believe that the core problem is that research in psychiatry is significantly under emphasized. This is the result of two misperceptions by psychiatrists: first, that we actually know enough about the disorders we treat, and second, that detailed knowledge about our target organ (the brain) is not necessary for effective practicing. The third problem is that the public believes that enough is known about the causes, diagnosis, and treatment of psychiatric disorders. These misconceptions conspire to decrease the public outcry for more research in psychiatry and decrease the desire of young psychiatrists to pursue research careers.

A major problem is the undue dependence on grants funding for the conduct of research. Junior research faculty have to work long hours juggling clinical, teaching, and administrative duties between grant deadlines, as well as enduring the repeated dismay with every grant rejection. Of course, the pay is not great either. No surprise then that not too many bright psychiatrists flock to this grinding machine. I once heard one of my most prominent professors using the term “disposable assistant professors” to describe young hopeful physicians aspiring to research careers who find themselves out of research opportunities once they have failed to secure funding for their projects.

Fundamental changes need to occur. Most important is the recognition that a monumental amount of research needs to be done before our understanding of psychiatric disorders is enough to allow predicting, preventing, effectively treating and rehabilitating patients. This goal cannot be met with the current dependence of research on National Institutes of Health (NIH), National Science Foundation (NSF), philanthropies, or industry funding. According to the NIMH website, the agency will target *schizophrenia, depression, suicide, autism,* bioterrorism and HIV. This is a small fraction of psychiatric disorders. The NIH funds approximately 20% of submitted grant proposals. Many of the non-funded proposals are important studies. What is needed, is a fundamental change that will allow all academic institutions to significantly contribute to research. This will require greater emphasis on research productivity for holding tenured positions in academic departments and that local and state governments help facilitate building research infrastructures.

Academic departments of psychiatry should have *a primary mission of advancing knowledge* both via research and teaching at the cutting edge of knowledge. It should be mandatory that psychiatry residents complete and publish a research project as part of the requirement for graduation. This will assure first hand knowledge of the actual mechanics of research as well as an advanced knowledge at least in one area of psychiatry. I would actually go further and propose that psychiatric residencies should be 5 years (it is now four years) with at least 18 months fully dedicated to research activities. The two fundamental points being made here are that undue dependence on NIH funding may indeed not be the most effective way of promoting research in psychiatry and that ways need to be found that will allow all academic departments of psychiatry to significantly contribute to psychiatric research.

The essential problem is the pervasive attitude that research is not of a paramount importance. Indeed, the overwhelming majority of academic departments of psychiatry in the US produce minimal research. Most residents graduate with no knowledge regarding research design, research conduct or the ethics of research. Many have no idea about what research careers are like. The problem stems from the fact that many chairs of academic departments of psychiatry are themselves not researchers. The position of Director of Residency hardly ever attracts serious researchers. It is thus no surprise that, with the exception of few noted research institutions, research is relegated to secondary if not lower status professionals, usually at significantly lower pay. Moreover, with many institutions doing away with the tenure system for clinical researchers, even this last attractive carrot is rapidly fading.

I think the institutions involved in mental health – the *American Psychiatric Association (APA)*, Consumer groups, and the National Institutes of Health (NIH) that are concerned with psychiatric disorders: the *National Institute of Mental Health (NIMH),* the National Institute on Drug Abuse (NIDA), and the National Institute on Alcohol, Alcohol Abuse and Alcoholism (NIAAA) – should develop a national policy where psychiatric research is considered an absolute priority. Everything else would likely follow.

Of course, it would be great if funding would be increased to train residents on research activity. This, on the other hand, is totally unnecessary for patient-oriented research learning. It may be necessary to educate our residents who may want to pursue more basic science research. To take example from my own work, I ran a very active clinical research team. Also, I ran a very active clinical care team. The two teams were completely separate. Residents did show some interest in knowing what we did in the lab (out of curiosity), but in the absence of a requirement and mandate it was simply more work for them. This attitude among psychiatry residents was most obvious during my last academic position when I was in fact the Department Chairperson. The minimal requirement of having each resident publish either a case report or a literature review during their four years of residency training was met with severe resistance. This was an amazing contrast as the pharmD residents had a similar requirement to be completed during one year only. To my knowledge, major Canadian academic departments have a five-year residency program. In these programs, residents spend at least 18 months in research activities. This is exactly what I propose here for our academic departments of psychiatry (all of them). Residents could complete their clinical requirements in the first 36 months and then focus on a research program of their choosing and in the area of their interest. This would actually be enough to encourage mentoring, as the mentors would claim academic credit for work performed by the residents. During the post-graduate years (PGY-IV & V) residents could function almost independently and should be able to generate their own salary needs. Many could also moonlight to generate additional personal income.

I also strongly recommend that every academic department to have a position for a Vice-Chair for research. This person would oversee the research training of the residents in his or her department. Waiting for funding is not the answer as money is short. Solutions can and must be found where research can be boosted with our currently available resources.

LEARNING THE LATEST

An absolutely essential learning skill is to get in the habit of checking the literature on a routine basis. This is a tall order as the number of journals with relevance to psychiatry is steadily rising with several dedicated to each one of the many disorders we deal with in this discipline. It is hard for me to accept a physician's claim that she/he is an expert in a certain disorder if he/she does not routinely read the relevant journals, belong to the national organization that has this focus, attend the annual meetings and perhaps other national or internationally relevant conferences.

Learning to Read Literature Critically

Furthermore, just reading the literature is not enough. Being able to critically read research publications as well as review articles, including meta-analyses, is an essential skill that will take concerted effort during residency and fellowship years to acquire. At least a small portion of research could be ill-motivated. Only an aware, skilled clinician will be able to avoid being influenced by such work (Vysohlid & Walton, 1990).

To develop this skill, the reader has to be reasonably familiar with the disorder being investigated, including what is known via available recent literature. This is essential as contradictory or unexpected claims warrant closer scrutiny. The reader must also have some basic knowledge of research designs as well as the proper statistics to be used with different data sets. Finally, the reader will only develop the sense of logic for the flow of the work from the introduction to the methods used and results to the conclusions derived from the results. It is not unusual that the conclusions reached by the investigators are completely unsupported by the findings, or less severely just out of proportion to the findings (Walton, 2001).

Research as Part of the Deal

Once a research culture and significant infrastructure are set, incorporating research into training programs becomes part of the course. Four elements are necessary for the development of an investigator: mentorship, clinical populations, laboratory space, and funds.

Mentorship is the most important ingredient of the process and the most difficult to come by. Thankfully, the recent advances in communication abilities like video conferencing, skyping, email and even cloud-based data storage allows effective long-distance mentoring. Long-distance mentoring does need to be fostered and encouraged so the few leading authorities can help develop many younger and productive investigators. Throughout my career I saw a major change where in the early stages (late last century) all mentoring was local. During the latter part of my career I was able to mentor residents/junior faculty across the globe.

Clinical populations are usually readily quite available in the communities where the teaching institutions exist but not in an organized enough fashion that allows easy incorporation into investigational endeavors. The development of specialized and sub-specialized clinics will readily allow such populations to be organized. This re-organization should not present the institutions with an additional burden. It is a matter of matching the diagnosis with the clinics. For example, if there is a "Thought-Disorders" Program, then one clinic could be dedicated to positive symptoms (e.g., hallucinations and delusions), one to deficit syndrome (patients with decreased affect and volition), and one to clozaril needing patients (usually difficult to treat schizophrenia patients). Another clinic would be dedicated to delusional disorder, one could be for schizoaffective disorder, and yet one more for those thought to have drug-induced psychosis. Such clinics would allow the routine use of standardized rating scales for all workers in the clinic (nurses, social workers, case managers) to develop special expertise in assessing and managing this particular problem. Once patients in a particular clinic are fully assessed, they are then available for inclusion in many subsequent projects. Some of these projects may have some funding attached as a bonus for the patients they represent.

Space is always available. As a matter of observation, there usually is a reciprocal relationship between the intensity of research in an institution and the availability of space. Furthermore, once an investigator has developed a functioning laboratory, the laboratory usually can perform many more studies utilizing the same space and equipment.

Finally, we come to the issue of funding. As I have argued repeatedly, when a city, county, or a state decides to establish a medical school, funds must be assigned for research in general and specifically for psychiatric research. Large hospitals that are university-affiliated must also work towards generating funds for research. One way I found possible was to develop “Faculty or Research Clinics” where a small surcharge is added to support research.

In conclusion, research is the only way forward for any branch of medicine but for psychiatry it is most indispensable and needs to simply be a part of what EVERY practitioner does on a routine basis. It follows that education regarding all aspects of research must be part of the education of psychiatry residents.

Chapter 8

RESEARCH IN PSYCHIATRY

NEED FOR MUCH MORE RESEARCH

The field of psychiatry is large. The DSM-5 lists over 120 disorders. Each one of these disorders is rather complex, diverse in character (i.e., heterogenous) with individuals often afflicted by more than one (i.e., comorbidity). The scope of research necessary to understand these disorders is huge and requires many investigators collaborating as well as extensive funding. Currently, research is being conducted in only a few institutions. The overwhelming majority of patients suffering from these disorders are treated in *community mental health centers* (CMHC) or by private practitioners whose data from everyday practice is not systematically collected or analyzed. In other words, experimentation is being conducted on a daily basis and the field is not benefitting from sharing the results.

Given the early nature of the field of biological psychiatry, all diagnostic and therapeutic activities can be seen as experimental. When a psychiatrist in a community mental health center makes a diagnosis, it is, indeed, an experiment as the test-retest reliability of the current diagnostic system is less than optimal or even desirable. Hence, the impact of accurate versus less then accurate or downright wrong diagnoses on the long-term management and outcome are not known. Similarly, when a psychiatrist prescribes a medication, it is also an experiment. At our current state of knowledge response to medication cannot be accurately predicted. Choice of medications remains a matter of the preference of the prescribing physician. Large scale efficacy studies are thus, in fact, being conducted on daily basis and we are deprived of learning the results of these experiments due to the lack of organization.

Based on humanistic ideals we propose that the entire discipline of psychiatry be declared a research enterprise. While this proposition would have been patently absurd only a few years back due to the lack of technology capable of linking up both institutions and physicians, this is a possibility in our current time. The best and already available example is the Veterans Administration healthcare system (VAHS). All of the VA hospitals' medical records are already linked nationwide, allowing investigators to mine extremely large amounts of data. Major changes to the current practice of psychiatry would need to be instituted, most importantly the standardization of clinical evaluation and the management of patients. The institution of standardized rating scales would go a long way towards achieving this goal. The switch from unstructured interaction with patients to semi-structured or completely structured interviews will immediately raise the standard of care. Medication choice algorithms are already available from a number of sources and could be instituted to provide guidance to the managing physician.

A substantial improvement in the level of awareness and knowledge of the practicing psychiatrists is sorely needed. Many practitioners are unable to recognize unusual or instructive cases when they come through their patient loads. Even if they realize that something is interesting and worth reporting in a case, having never done so (i.e., submitted a case report for peer review for publication) is a prohibitive obstacle. This sort of effort is seen as a waste of valuable time unless a way to incentivize such activity is developed. We must assume that many such cases are routinely missed to the detriment of the field. In fact, in many CMHCs or private clinics return visits are sometimes allowed less than 15 minutes. New evaluations may be allowed 45 minutes, such time allotments are hardly enough for thorough evaluations let alone consideration of interesting aspects of the cases. The above proposals would indeed take many years and concerted effort in order to commence and it would be natural that it would be met with much resistance.

GLOBALIZATION OF RESEARCH

All what was said regarding US psychiatry applies to rest of the world. In fact, much research that is conducted and reported in non-English Language journals is unknown to English speaking investigators who are thus likely to replicate it without the benefit of already conducted studies (Boutros N, 2013). Some form of global organization of psychiatric research must be created. There are already a number of organizations that can immediately be thought of as possible avenues for such activity. First, the World Health Organization (WHO) has already active organs in all areas of the world, including far removed regions where the conduct of research could be extremely informative to rest of the world and would help transform the clinical care provided in those particular regions. The World Psychiatric Association (WPA) and the World Federation of Societies of Biological Psychiatry (WFSBP) can and must also play major roles in integrating world efforts to achieve the above goals.

Translational Research; Lets Link the Ivory Tower to the Practicing Clinicians

Medication development research should go to universities. I have usually practiced in inner-city situations, where it is an everyday occurrence that one patient cannot afford the medication prescribed by the treating psychiatrist. While less desirable alternatives that are more affordable can usually be found, it is fundamentally unfair as this only affects the poor and disadvantaged. It is thus of paramount importance that newly discovered psychiatric medications be reasonably priced right from the outset. The story of clozapine, the medication used to treat *Scizophrenia,* was particularly revealing. Upon the release of clozapine, the cost of treatment was usually borne out by family members in cash and at close to one thousand dollars per month. Obviously, many patients who needed to be on clozapine were not able to receive it until many years later. Under humanistic psychiatry, this would be entirely unacceptable. Allen Frances in his masterful book "Saving Normal" sounds a loud alarm regarding the role of the pharmaceutical industry in corrupting American Psychiatry and asks for strong control over their activity. It is sad that the US is the only industrialized nation that allows direct advertising to the consumers. Here we strongly argue that the role of developing new treatments (including medications) should be an academic effort lead by academic institutions.

Supporting industry: The development of new psychiatric medications should not be a capitalist venture but a scientific endeavor. Nonetheless, major academic institutions that take this task on must be able to recoup their costs, including faculty support and education occurring in the process. Industry will remain involved but mainly in the production and marketing end of the process after academic institutions have developed and tested the drugs.

Translating Biological Parameters into Clinically-Useful Diagnostic Tests

Currently psychiatry does not have laboratory measures to serve as diagnostic tests or even to screen for possible disorders. As an essential part of modern medicine, laboratory tests are used to confirm, provide supportive evidence, rule out diagnoses, and follow up of the progression of the disorder. As a screener, the tests would highlight those individuals who should receive a more detailed assessment for a definitive diagnosis.

The lack of such measures in psychiatry cannot be attributed to the lack of candidates. Biological research into the pathophysiology of psychiatric disorders has yielded a number of highly replicable abnormalities which have the potential for being developed into clinically useful laboratory tests. One example is the P300 amplitude abnormalities in schizophrenia (Jeon and Polich, 2003). The P300 is an evoked electrical brain response that can be measured at the scalp. Despite the fact that this abnormality has been replicated in upward of 140 well-designed studies from laboratories around the world, studies specifically designed to translate the findings into diagnostic tests are sorely needed. Complicating the picture, these same abnormalities are also used to define endophenotypes (de Wilde et al. 2008). An endophenotype is a biological change that is linked to a disorder and can be used for genetic studies. How endophenotypes differ from diagnostic tests has not been clarified. The challenge is to efficiently bridge the vast gulf between biological research and clinical applications.

Although this challenge is not unique to psychiatry, the lack of current laboratory measures for diagnoses underscores the difficulty in translating biological research into clinical applications. In the past, laboratory tests were disseminated prior to rigorous testing to determine their clinical utility. The failure of the tests to match their marketed expectation meant disappointment and perhaps premature abandonment of the tests (Mokhtari et al. 2012). Even worse, if tests are used out of context, they may hinder the diagnostic and treatment process and increase overall costs.

Previous research into the readiness for biological abnormalities to be tested diagnostically (Boutros et al. 2008) revealed a substantial body of literature documenting the existence of abnormalities in some patient populations compared to normal controls. However, there remains a scant literature to move the results towards being test ready. By looking at the research literature using standardized categories, the need for certain types of research can be easily highlighted.

The development of laboratory diagnostic procedures is an essential step to help the field move forward as diagnosis in psychiatry remains a major limiting step in clinical studies (van Praag, 1997). While substantial work has been done investigating endophenotypes as a way to decrease the heterogeneity of the diagnoses, less attention has been paid to the use of laboratory tests as a way to improve diagnoses. To promote a standard approach, we proposed a four-step process for developing laboratory-based tests for use in aiding the diagnostic process in psychiatry (Boutros et al. 2008). In this chapter, we expand on these steps to incorporate existing processes for reporting diagnostic tests (STARD, Bruns 2005), developing guidelines (Appraisal of Guidelines for Research Evaluation or AGREE, Bussuyt et al. 2003) and evaluating evidence-based medicine (e.g., AGREE, 2003). We also contrast diagnostic tests with endophenotypes as biological investigators may focus their research on defining endophenotypes as opposed to developing diagnostic tests.

Each step will be briefly summarized and then augmented with input from the other fields. Finally, the contrast between endophenotypes and diagnostic tests will be summarized.

Step 1

In Step 1, a biological variable is observed to be deviant from healthy controls in a particular patient population. This initial step is necessary but not sufficient for a diagnostic test. The demonstration of test-retest reliability of the finding using masked (i.e., blinding of either investigators, patients or both) procedures is an essential component of this early step. Thus, there needs to be replication of the masked finding by the same or collaborating groups. However, confirmation by independent groups is essential for this particular test to move into the next step of development. As investigators may significantly influence other groups of investigators (e.g., via mentoring or teaching), it is vital that the replicating group be truly independent. In order to consider a group independent, there should be no common co-authors to the original description nor should they be from the same institution or be former mentees. Ideally, more than one independent replication should be required as the initial results may be context- or patient selection-specific. The greater difference in geographic settings for the replications, the greater the confidence in the generalizability of the biological difference. However, this latter criterion is problematic as it is more difficult to have replications published, particularly in the more prestigious journals. This step can be summarized as providing evidence of consistent biological abnormality in the target population.

The AGREE criteria argue more forcefully than we had previously that the independence of researchers also includes independence of financial ties to potential developers of the technology. Thus, even at Step 1 it is important to examine conflicts of interest and to assure other researchers and clinicians that the biological abnormality is not conveniently found and replicated for fiduciary gain.

The STARD criteria further require that the abnormality and means to test it be fully described so that it can be readily replicated. This requires full disclosure of the recruitment process, of other conditions present (e.g., are smokers allowed in the normal controls?), and that it be tested in both genders and in minorities. For statistical comparison, the actual descriptive statistics (e.g., means and standard deviations) are needed as opposed to just stating whether the results were significant or non-significant.

Step 2

Step 2 is the demonstration of the potential clinical usefulness of the specific finding found and replicated in Step 1. The objective at this step is to demonstrate consistent difference between the target patient population and groups of patients with closely related diagnoses. Closely related diagnoses would be disorders that commonly appear on the differential diagnostic lists of the target disorder. Instead of documenting a difference between target patients and healthy controls, this step requires the biological abnormality to be *specific* to the target population and not occur in phenomenologically similar patients. This specificity is important as an abnormality that is equally common to disorders that need to be differentiated from one another (e.g., Bipolar Disorder and Schizophrenia) is not likely to be useful clinically. Abnormalities with significant differential prevalence among disorders to be differentiated are needed to confirm, provide supportive information for, or rule out a diagnosis. However, biological abnormalities may not offer clear evidence of specificity but offer some additional information. In this case, the cost of the test, burden on the patients and implications of incorrect diagnoses need to be evaluated. This step is consistent with AGREE, STARD and evidence-based medicine criteria that the target patients with the abnormality are specifically described and those not targeted are described. It also is consistent with evidence-based medicine criteria that the tests be conducted in an appropriate spectrum of patients that clinicians would likely encounter in their practices.

Step 3

During Step 3, the performance characteristics of the test should be established. At this stage the sensitivity, specificity, and positive and negative predictive values of the biological marker should be examined. These data should allow the estimation of the added diagnostic value resulting from incorporating the test into the work-up of a particular patient. The choice of the "gold standard" or reference test is an essential component of this step. This is the standard against which the test being developed will be measured. The currently accepted gold standard in psychiatric diagnosis is the *Best Estimate Diagnosis* (Kosten & Rounsaville, 1992). The Best Estimate Diagnosis is the agreement between experts based upon the data available. The data could include longitudinal observations and reports from family, work, or school. It may also include standardized scales or tasks with demonstrated reliability and validity. One difficulty with this approach is that diagnostic classifications may change in the future. In this situation, a biological abnormality that does not distinguish between clinically similar patients may offer etiological clues and may be useful for future diagnostic classifications.

At this step, the clinical characteristics of the patient group identified by the test are usually further delineated. Due to the heterogeneous nature of psychiatric disorders, it would be unreasonable to expect any one biological test to be able to identify all patients that are classified into a current disorder category (e.g., schizophrenia). It is much more likely that a particular test will be able to identify one or more sub-groups within these categories. Defining the clinical characteristics of the sub-group that is identifiable by a particular test would be very important for the test to be considered for clinical use. Factors such as effects of illness duration and severity and the effects of medications should also be defined during this stage (AGREE, 2003). The biological abnormality may also predict prognosis. The step could include a variety of study designs, excluding multicenter clinical trials needed to confirm the diagnostic utility of the biological abnormality. The standardization of the tests is further refined at this stage.

From evidence-based medicine and STARD we know that a test must be demonstrated to be sensitive and specific. This information, however, is not sufficient to recommend the biological abnormality as a diagnostic test. Even though our previous review of EEG (brain wave test) abnormalities in schizophrenia found few Step 3 studies (Boutros et al. 2008), they are more prevalent in other fields. For example, PSA was advocated to screen for prostate cancer based upon multiple Step 3 studies. Unfortunately, the recent publications of two independent clinical trials (what we call Step 4, described below) failed to confirm the usefulness of PSA as a screener (Andriole et al. 2009; Schroder et al. 2009).

Step 4

Step 4 defines the clinical application of the test and standardizes the technique through the use of multicenter clinical trials. Multicenter trials are needed to standardize laboratory procedures, collect data of cost effectiveness, and document impact on short-term and long-term clinical outcomes. Studies in earlier steps depend on smaller samples of control subjects that are usually locally formed. On the other hand, Step 4 studies provide data collected using a defined protocol over greater geographic and clinical context with a growing diversity of patients (e.g., with multiple disorders). These data *prove* the clinical utility and contribute to establishing norms against which clinicians can compare values for a specific patient. The four steps are summarized below in Table 1.

Table 1. Summary of the four steps proposed to developing diagnostic tests in Psychiatry

Step	Design	Purposes	Desired Outcomes
1	Target group vs. healthy controls	1) Demonstration of significant deviance in the target group. 2) Demonstration of test- retest reliability of finding.	Provide evidence of a consistent biological abnormality in the target group.
2	Target group vs. healthy and appropriate patient control groups.	Demonstration of significant differential prevalence of abnormality between illnesses that frequently need to be differentiated from one another.	Demonstration of potential clinical utility.
3	Target vs. proper control groups (may include within target group sub-populations.	Definition of test-performance characteristics.	Defining clinical utility.
4	Same as in Step 3 but across centers, ideally in a multicenter design.	Demonstration and standardization of clinical application.	Setting up standards for clinical application.

As mentioned in Step 2, it is not expected that biological abnormalities will be sufficient to diagnose one specific disorder. Instead, they are expected to contribute independent information as part of an overall assessment of the individual. As part of STARD criteria, it is important that the specific contribution of the abnormality be defined. Consistent with *evidence-based* medicine criteria, the test must be affordable and useful in the setting of the clinician. It must add information that affects clinical management.

These four steps are presented as a way to classify the research requirements for the development of a diagnostic test or screener. In this way, policy makers can point to the inadequacy in existing research findings on specific biological abnormalities using the broad outline of steps. The recent failure in multicenter clinical trials of PSA as a screener for prostate cancer underscores the necessity of including all four steps in a strategy to develop tests or screeners. However, when examining specific abnormalities, there is clearly the need to include costs, patients' preferences, clinical practicality of the tests, and the implications of potentially wrong diagnoses in determining if the biological phenomena should be translated into diagnostic tests.

We present the steps also as way to classify existing literature. Our previous reviews have found an abundance of Step 1 studies, some Step 2 studies and very few Step 3 studies (Boutros et al. 2008). Step 4 studies were conspicuously absent. To propel the development of diagnostic tests, more focused funding and research is needed. This research needs to be consistent with the principles of *evidence-based* medicine and can be informed by criteria developed by other groups.

Finally, there have been extensive discussions and a growing amount of literature on endophenotypes. Diagnostic tests clearly are distinct from developing endophenotypes (Table 2). For the biological abnormality to qualify for consideration for a diagnostic test, it must be specific to one disorder. Such specificity is in sharp contrast to endophenotypes which by their definition are examining specific genetic vulnerability and can be useful for redefining disorders. To move psychiatry forward, research addressing both diagnostic tests and endophenotypes are needed.

Table 2. Differences between Endophenotypes and Diagnostic Tests

Endophenotypes	**Diagnostic Tests**
Must be in the majority of patients with the target disorder	Must be in the majority of patients with the target disorder
Must be trait and not state dependent	Can be state or trait dependent
Must be seen in non-ill family members	Should not be present in non-ill individuals (but can be present at less than diagnostic levels)
Required to be heritable	Not required to be heritable
Can be present in related disorders	Must be significantly less prevalent in related disorders

THE NIH AND THE NATIONAL PSYCHIATRY RESEARCH EFFORT

Do the National Institutes of Health (NIH) that are mainly concerned with psychiatry: *National Institute of Mental Health* (NIMH), National Institute of Drug Abuse (NIDA), and the National Institute of Alcohol Alcoholism and Alcohol Use (NIAAA) facilitate or hinder psychiatric research? I believe this is a question worth asking.

The initial premise I would like to start with is that research will and does go on with or without the support of NIH or the National Science Foundation (NSF). The question that has arisen recently in the current environment of almost impossible funding, is whether the current set up and procedures for obtaining NIH funding is hurting psychiatric research.

Let me begin by stating why I think this may be the case. The most serious damage occurs when young, bright physicians turn away from research as they see the suffering of mid-level MD-investigators or even well-established professors. Many a time a resident wanders into my office at 7 or 8 PM seeing me working on a Saturday or Sunday and finding me glued to my computer. They always ask what am I doing there and the answer is always, "Working on a grant." They then ask, "Well, Dr. Boutros, how many grants do you have and how many do you need?" They then are utterly surprised to learn that I am about to become an unfunded investigator when my last RO1 (the most common form of grants funded by the NIH) expires. Frequently, they feel bad for me and pull up a chair and begin to want to know more about academia.

It is a fact that successful academicians are self motivated and driven. This is good news because it means that most of the individuals in this breed will go on and become researchers. The bad news is that some will be driven away. In my opinion, we cannot afford to lose these.

Why Intramural NIH Research?

After exhausting search I am yet to find evidence that research conducted intramurally at any of the psychiatry-related institutes (NIMH, NIDA, NIAAA) is superior to research conducted by any of the leading research universities. By doing away with intramural funding and the huge bureaucracy that goes with it, the NIH would be able to support much more research in many universities currently starved for funding.

Why Does the NIH Not Follow Careers of Individuals on Tenure Tracks??

When physicians decide to dedicate their careers to research, they usually make a significant financial sacrifice. Salaries in very prestigious institutions are consistently significantly lower than in comparable private practice settings. Many such physicians are being taken advantage off as they are driven to work in suboptimal situations and for long hours without much research support or guidance.

The proposal here is that the NIH approves all tenure track positions and monitor and support all such faculty and be an integral part of negotiating their packages and judging their promotions. It may follow that universities will be afforded a certain number of tenure track slots for developing research in the institution based on the investment from the university and the state or the city where the institution happens to be.

Tenure-track positions should be regulated by the NIH and supported by the cities/states where the institutions are. Recruiting bright young MDs to the field of psychiatry research is an uphill battle for an academic institution without huge name recognition. While recruiting such scholars at Yale or Johns Hopkins is usually not very hard, it is almost impossible to recruit such individuals to universities like the one where I was the Chairperson in Kansas City, Missouri. Incorporating research support and protected research time into such positions will facilitate this process. It remains that proper and effective mentorship must be assured. Nowadays and thanks to the fast and effective communication abilities, mentorship can be performed long-distance. Either the candidate faculty member identifies a mentor or the NIH can do that. Mentors' performances can be evaluated based on feedback from mentees. ONLY selected physicians with proven productivity and commitment to the field should be able to compete for these positions and clear guidelines for maintaining the position or getting promoted must be developed.

In other words, the NIMH/NIDA/NIAAA must not be "research Institutions" but rather institutions that monitor and guide research across the entire country. It just strikes me as hugely unjust to require a researcher in a much less powerful and established research institution to compete with a researcher from a prestigious university for an RO1. As funding is seen by funding institutions (all of them) as investments, the name and track record of the fund-requesting institution play major roles (the so-called funding by zip codes). The fact is that many excellent grant proposals go unfunded for the simple reason of lack of money!!!!

Chapter 9

PERSONALITY DISORDERS

INTRODUCTION

Personality disorders are the remaining frontier where the disorders remain mysterious and the question of whether they are real disorders or just extremes of normal ranges of behavior still lurks in the discussion. While much research has been dedicated to some disorders in this group, most notably borderline personality disorder (BPD) and antisocial personality disorder (APD), most of the other personality disorders received much less research emphasis. In particular, the neurobiological underpinnings of Narcissistic, Dependent, Schizoid, or Obsessive-Compulsive Personality Disorders remain largely unknown. One factor that perhaps has played a role in this de-emphasis is that this group of disorders is not included among what are called "severe and persistent mental illness (SMI)." In fact, most of the afflicted individuals endure suffering while trying to navigate life, not understanding why their lives must be so difficult. Vazquez et al, (2017) challenged the concept of SMI.

They evaluated the clinical severity as well as healthcare spending on dissociative disorders (DDs). A member of this group of disorders is multiple personality disorder (MPD).

This diagnostic group was compared with two other groups usually considered as causes of severe impairment and high healthcare spending: psychotic disorders including bipolar disorder, and unipolar depression. From a random sample of 200 psychiatric outpatients, 108 with unipolar depression (N = 45), psychotic/bipolar (N = 31) or DDs (N = 32) were selected for this study. The three groups were compared by the severity of their disorders and healthcare indicators. Of the three groups, those with a DD were more prone to and showed higher indices of suicide, self-injury, emergency consultations, as well as psychotropic drug use. This group ranked just below psychotic/bipolar patients in the number/duration of psychiatric hospitalizations. While there is a lack of similar studies addressing other personality, anxiety, or substance use disorders, there are no reasons to consider such disorders less serious.

Personality disorders are not less stigmatizing. Perhaps the most stigmatizing diagnosis among all psychiatric disorders is anti-social personality disorder (see more detail in the chapter on "Correctional Psychiatry") but with borderline personality not far behind. With such stigma attached to these disorders, patients not only resist and resent the diagnosis; they also are highly unlikely to seek help unless forced into it. There is no doubt that more research is needed in this much less evolved sub-field of Psychiatry.

Biological Principle Has to Be Applied

The enduring and frequently devastating effects of these disorders on the individuals' lives is such that biological brain deviations must play a major role. In fact, accumulating evidence is clearly pointing in this direction. Below we review some of the evidence but by no means provide a comprehensive review of this slowly expanding literature.

Researchers typically analyze samples of pairs of twins in order to decompose trait variance into genetic and environmental components. This methodological technique, referred to as twin-based research, rests on several assumptions that must be satisfied in order to produce unbiased results. Jang (2013) describes a major and ongoing effort at the University of British Columbia to answer this question. The question of the relative contribution of genetics vs environmental factors remains not fully answered (Barnes & Boutwell, 2013). In a recent set of data from children, psychopathic personality traits were assessed in a total of 1189 5-year-old boys and girls drawn from the Preschool Twin Study in Sweden. Psychopathic personality traits were assessed with the Child Problematic Traits Inventory, a teacher-reported measure of psychopathic personality traits in children ranging from 3 to 12 years old. Univariate results showed that genetic influences accounted for 57, 25, and 74% of the variance in the grandiose-deceitful, callous-unemotional, and impulsive-need for stimulation dimensions, respectively. These results are statistically significant. The shared environment accounted for 17, 48 and 9% in grandiose-deceitful and callous-unemotional, impulsive-need for stimulation dimensions, respectively. No sex differences were found in the genetic and environmental variance components. The non-shared environment accounted for the remaining 26, 27 and 17% of the variance, respectively. The three dimensions of psychopathic personality were moderately correlated (0.54-0.66) and these correlations were primarily mediated by genetic and shared environmental factors (Tuvblad et al. 2017).

The case is a bit clearer for Borderline Personality Disorder (BPD). Familial and twin studies largely support the potential role of a genetic vulnerability at the root of BPD, with an estimated heritability of approximately 40%. Moreover, there is evidence for both gene-environment interactions and correlations. However, association studies for BPD are sparse, making it difficult to draw clear conclusions (Amad et al. 2014). Research on the genetics of other personality disorders is even more sparse. Gjerde et al. (2015) provided evidence that phenotypic stability was moderate for both avoidant and obsessive-compulsive personality disorders traits, and that genetic factors contributed more than unique environmental factors to the stability both within and across phenotypes. The inescapable conclusion is that significantly more research remains necessary to elucidate the balance between genetic and environmental contributions to these life-long disorders.

Early Identification, Education, Support and Treatment

Given the highly stigmatizing nature of the disorders, efforts towards early detection are likely to be resisted. ONLY when the disorders are de-stigmatized and the public, particularly schools, are educated about them, will we be able to begin to try programs for early detection. As with any ailment known to humankind, early intervention, including education and support, is likely to yield better results than late intervention.

As is repeatedly asserted in this book, the "Brain" is the only way out of stigma. By being able to identify the biological underpinning of these disorders, we can begin to discuss them as real disorders and plan for the early detection, intervention and rehabilitation.

While I am not aware of studies attempting prevention of BPD, there have been serious attempts at preventing APD (Waddell et al, 1999). Based on the knowledge that APD takes its roots in childhood and that the syndrome never breaks in a full-blown picture, attempts at early detection and working with children as they exhibit the early signs of deviation had had some success, despite being limited overall (Kazdin & Durbin, 2012). Nonetheless, studies concluded that the advantages of preventing antisocial behavior before it gathers momentum and becomes established are overwhelming. The evidence to date suggests that concerted community as well as targeted efforts need to be combined to improve the chances of success. What is most encouraging is that when intervention is instituted prior to the diagnosis, to a major degree it avoids the stigma and the possible harmful effects of the diagnosis.

Some Selected Evidence for the Biological Nature of the Two Most Stigmatizing and Most Studied Personality Disorders

Borderline personality disorder (BPD) patients constitute a large burden on the resources of mental health services. Developing a thorough understanding of the neurobiology of BPD is essential for the development of effective preventive, therapeutic, and rehabilitative approaches to the disorder. Although BPD is one of the most investigated of the personality disorders, the neurobiological bases of the disorder remain largely unknown. Evidence for an organic basis for BPD has been forthcoming since the 1980s. Efforts to bring rapidly advancing neuro-investigative technology to bear on the understanding of this disorder is likely to contribute significantly to the unraveling of the underlying pathophysiological processes and the identification of any biological subtypes this disorder might have.

A number of electrophysiological studies linked BPD to complex partial seizures (CPSs) (Muller, 1992). Andrulonis et al. (1982) found that 27% of adolescent BPD patients had evidence of brain dysfunction or current epilepsy. They also found history of head trauma, encephalitis, or past seizures in 11%. Several episodic or paroxysmal symptoms are common between BPD and temporal lobe epilepsy complex partial seizures (CPS): impulsivity, transient psychosis, and intermittent experience of depersonalization (abnormal sensations of one's own body parts) and derealization (abnormal perceptions in the environment) (Fenwick, 1981. Carbamazepine (a commonly used seizure medication) has been shown to be effective in decreasing paroxysmal symptoms (Cowdry & Gardner, 1988). Indeed, a number of case reports have described CPSs in patients who had previously been diagnosed with BPD (Messner, 1986, Schmidt et al. 1989). In a separate set of reports, BPD has been linked to affective/mood disorders (Perry, 1985). A high rate of co-occurring depressive symptoms among BPD patients has long been observed. Indeed, longitudinal studies have found that even cases of apparently pure BPD, when followed over time, are characterized by frequent suicide attempts and clear-cut affective episodes (Pope et al. 1983). In a third branch of the literature, BPD has been linked to psychotic disorders (Gunderson et al. 1981; Schultz et al. 1988). The partial clinical response among BPD patients to antipsychotic agents further supports a possible relationship to psychotic disorders (Brinkley et al. 1979; Soloff et al. 1981).

In a review of the then available literature, Korzekwa et al. (1993) suggested that BPD is an independent disorder with at least two possible biological subtypes: an affective subtype and a psychotic subtype. Coccaro and Kavoussi (1991) suggested that the identification of such subtypes can be useful in guiding treatment choices. A better understanding of electrophysiological as well as other biological abnormalities in BPD would also facilitate the examination of the relationship between abnormalities related to child abuse and those identified in adult patients.

Child abuse has been shown to result in clinical electroencephalogram (EEG) (Rosenberg et al, 2000), as well as other measurable brain electrical signal abnormalities (Ito et al. 1988). Child abuse has been strongly linked to the development of BPD (Zanarini et al. 1997). Electrophysiological as well as structural and functional brain imaging technologies have rapidly advanced in the past two decades. Computerized quantification of electroencephalography with the use of high-density electrode arrays has made it capable of accurate localization of the cerebral sources of scalp-recorded activity. The technology for recording and analyzing sleep (polysomnography) and cerebral evoked potentials (EPs) have similarly advanced, allowing more detailed examination of these biological signals. Moreover, newer, powerful techniques such as magnetoencephalography (MEG), which is capable of examining the magnetic brain signals (similar to the EEG signal but much smaller in magnitude) emanating from deeper cortical tissue, and transcranial magnetic stimulation (TMS), capable of non-invasively examining the excitability characteristics of the cortex in awake, behaving humans, have yet to be applied to the investigation of BPD. In order to assess the value and possible future contribution of electrophysiological investigative techniques, we examined the literature in which at least one of these techniques was used to examine patients with BPD (Boutros et al. 2005). The inescapable conclusion was that the plethora of readily identifiable abnormalities awaits well-designed studies to assess their diagnostic and prognostic clinical values as well as the possible impact on therapy choices.

ANTI-SOCIAL PERSONALITY DISORDER (ASPD)

EEG and Antisocial Personality Disorder

As early as the mid-1940s, it was recognized that criminals had a higher prevalence of EEG abnormalities. Among psychiatric populations the group of ''psychopaths' had the largest incidence of either borderline or frank abnormalities which consisted mainly of diffuse background slowing (un-medicated patients) and/or paroxysmal (epilepsy suggestive) activity (Hill and Watterson, 1942). Hill and Watterson (1942) examined the EEGs of 151 subjects with psychopathic personalities. They reported 48% of this group to exhibit abnormal *EEGs* as compared to 15% of a non-patient control group. When they divided the group into aggressive (N = 66) and nonaggressive, they found 65% of aggressive patients and only 32 % of nonaggressive subjects to exhibit abnormal EEGs. In this chapter, they also reported a significant relationship between a history of head injury and the presence of EEG abnormalities. They concluded that the more aggressive the patient the more likely the EEG to be abnormal. Wong et al. (1994) retrospectively examined the EEGs and CAT scans of 372 male patients in a maximum security mental hospital. Reviewers were blind to the specific history of the individual. They reported that 20% of the EEGs (and 41% of CAT scans) were abnormal in the most violent patients, as compared to 2.4 % (6.7% for CAT scans) for the least violent patients. Patients diagnosed with antisocial personality disorder frequently harbor organic brain pathology that can be assessed with the help of the EEG, along with other neuro-evaluative tools. Blake et al. (1995) performed detailed and thorough neurological evaluations of 31 individuals awaiting trial or sentencing for murder. EEGs, MRIs or CAT scans, and neuropsychological testing were obtained from most of the subjects. Neurological examination revealed evidence of ''frontal'' lobes dysfunction in 20 (64.5%). There were symptoms or some other evidence of temporal lobe dysfunction in 9 (29%). Specific neurologic diagnoses were made in 20 (64.5%). These diagnoses included borderline or full mental retardation in nine and cerebral palsy in two. Most importantly, neuropsychological testing of patients with episodic aggression and impulse dyscontrol (behaving normally most of the time but exhibiting unpredictable aggressive episodes) revealed abnormalities in all subjects tested. There were EEG abnormalities in eight of the 20 subjects who had EEGs. EEG abnormalities consisted mainly of bilateral epileptic activity and other abnormalities indicating brain tissue damage. There were MRI or CAT scans abnormalities in nine of 19 subjects tested, primarily atrophy and white matter changes. There was a documented history of profound and protracted physical abuse in 26 (83.8%) and sexual abuse in 10 (32.3%). They concluded that prolonged, severe physical abuse and neurological brain dysfunction interact with paranoia (all subjects had evidence of paranoid ideations) to form the matrix of violent behavior. It has also been shown that among groups of prisoners convicted of murder, the highest incidence of EEG abnormalities (74%) occurred in individuals whose crimes were apparently motiveless or had minimal motives (Stafford-Clark and Taylor 1949). A well-designed relatively large study of 265 consecutive admissions to a special hospital for offenders supported the above findings (Howard 1984). One of the major findings was that the prevalence of abnormalities was not different between medicated and unmedicated subjects, strongly suggesting that abnormalities in this population are not secondary to medication effects (64.8% for medicated and 61.4% for un-medicated patients). Secondly, at least full 50% of the subjects had clear EEG abnormalities. This, indeed, seems to be the overall impression one gets from examining this complex body of literature. The close to 50% prevalence of EEG abnormalities in association with violence seems to be culturally independent. Okasha et al. (1975) reported a prevalence of 43 % of EEG abnormalities in a group of Egyptian murderers. Nelson and Boutros (1993) examined consecutive admissions to an inpatient adult psychiatry unit with diagnosis of antisocial personality and found the majority to have evidence of organic brain involvement (majority with EEG abnormalities) warranting changing the diagnosis in a majority of subjects to Organic Personality Disorder according to the DSM-III.

The thorough understanding of the biological mechanisms contributing to habitual aggression is fundamental if effective preventive, diagnostic, and rehabilitative programs are to be developed. Electrophysiological techniques, including conventional and quantified EEG, can be very helpful in advancing our knowledge of this area. Of great interest is the serious gap between a large body of literature attesting to the prevalence of neuropsychological, electrophysiological, and both structural and functional brain imaging abnormalities, and the actual utilization of this information in diagnosing and managing individuals exhibiting such symptoms. Moreover, the slow pace of more recent research in this area further widens this gap.

Episodic Aggression and Impulse Dyscontrol

As individuals with this condition are by definition normal between episodes and tend to be remorseful regarding any problems or damage they may have caused during an attack, they tend to not be included in ASPD studies by careful investigators. The prevalence of abnormal EEGs in this clinical population varies widely among studies ranging from as low as 6.6% in patients with rage attacks and episodic violent behavior (Riley and Niedermeyer 1978) to as high as 53% in patients diagnosed with antisocial personality disorder (Harper et al. 1972). Rare negative studies, showing lack of significant EEG abnormalities in patients with rage attacks or episodic violent behavior have also appeared. Bach-Y-Rita et al. (1971) reported the EEGs of 79 patients diagnosed with "episodic dyscontrol." Thirty-seven of them were abnormal (close to the widely reported 50% incidence). Of the 37 abnormal records, 20 showed epileptic activity in the temporal region. They classified patients who were included in the study into four categories; (1) patients already diagnosed with temporal lobe epilepsy; (2) patients with epilepsy like episodes; (3) patients with "diffuse violence" with violent outbursts at varied targets. These subjects constituted the largest group and exhibited a significantly increased level of anxiety. The fourth group was that with "pathological intoxication."

Bennett et al. (1983) examined the EEGs of 48 children between the ages of 5.2 and 12.9 years who were hospitalized for aggressive, explosive, or conduct disorders. EEGs were examined at baseline, on placebo, haloperidol, or lithium. They reported a prevalence of 58.3% abnormalities at baseline. Both haloperidol (an antipsychotic agent) and lithium (a mood-stabilizing agent) caused the EEGs to look more abnormal (even in children who seemed to be responding to treatment). It should be noted that three EEGs that were found to be normal on initial testing were found to be abnormal on subsequent testing later on while patients were on placebo. This finding attests to the value of repeated EEG testing.

Boelhouwer et al. (1968) was able to predict the presence of the 14 and 6 Positive Spikes (PS) by selecting a group of adolescents and young adults who exhibited episodic aggressive outbursts. The PS EEG pattern is a controversial one that is not believed to be related to epilepsy but is more commonly associated with what is called "vegetative behavior." Patients usually have multiple complaints and tend to have less impulse control. Subjects with PS had significantly higher histories of their mothers experiencing toxemia during pregnancy with them. With extensive psychological testing the PS individuals had significantly more problems with judgment and success of control mechanisms. It is of interest to note that these investigators found the PS to occur independently of any diagnostic category listed by the American Psychiatric Association at that time. Furthermore, subjects with PS had significantly more *anxiety* and were more insightful and more ready to feel guilty and be self-critical than subjects in a control group with similar behaviors but without PS. The treatment implications of these psychological findings were not discussed but a pharmacological investigation was reported. The study had a maximum of 8-week trials comparing thioridazine (antipsychotic), diphenylhydantoin (antiseizure), or combination of the two against a placebo. They reported that the PS group responded best to the combination of drugs. Monroe (1989) followed 50 patients with episodic dyscontrol or other episodic symptoms for 38 to 57 months. On the bases of alpha chloralose activated EEG results (an EEG activating procedure that is no longer in use), an anticonvulsant was recommended for 39 patients. Twenty patients received medications that raised the seizure threshold. Of these 20 patients, 10 reported marked and six reported moderate improvement.

Habitual Versus Sporadic Aggression

Williams (1969) compared the EEGs of 206 habitual aggressors and 127 who committed isolated acts of violence. He reported a five-fold increase in EEG abnormalities in habitual aggressors; 57% as compared to 21% in non-habitual aggressors. They also found more frontal region abnormalities in the habitual aggressors but more diffuse (wide spread) and epileptic activity in the non-habitual aggressors. Another important finding reported by Howard (1984) is that patients who had committed violent offences against strangers, as opposed to people known to them, tended to have bilateral EEG features suggestive of epilepsy; 70% of subjects with such abnormalities have attacked strangers.

The above limited review underscores two major facts. First, personality disorders are complex phenomena with identifiable biological deviations that are likely to eventually help identify diagnostically and therapeutically meaningful subtypes. Secondly, the volume of research needed to fully understand the various disorders must be many folds greater than the currently supported research effort.

Chapter 10

DRUG AND ALCOHOL USE DISORDERS

INTRODUCTION

At the outset, we must differentiate between occasional recreational use of any mind-altering drug where there is no evidence that a disorder exists and situations where drug use has demonstrable harmful consequences. This is crucially important to avoid a moral judgment on those who use drugs recreationally.

It is thus also paramount that objective biological diagnostic procedures be developed for both assessing increased risk to developing an addiction disorder as well as biological markers for when a disorder has, in fact, developed. This is important to avoid judgment diagnoses, over-diagnosing and stigmatizing individuals who may not in fact be suffering from a brain disorder. There is no way to avoid the existence of a grey zone between disorder and non-disease states as all human ailments tend to come in various degrees of severity with the mildest forms being the most difficult to differentiate from a healthy state. At this border area a huge inter-individual variability exists further complicating the issue. Here a combination of biological testing, clinical data, and biostatistics can help guide the decision-making process. In the "Research" chapter we propose and detail a 4-step approach to developing promising biological findings into clinically useful laboratory diagnostic tests.

Substance Abuse/Dependence Is a Brain Disorder

The evidence has now accumulated that clearly describes the brain circuitry dysfunction that helps perpetuate the abuse/dependence behavior. The reward circuitry is now well-characterized with the nucleus accumbens (a small structure deep within the brain) at its core. The role of dopamine as a reward neurotransmitter has also been elucidated. Nonetheless, it is the recent accumulated work of Nora Volkow (currently head of the National Institute on Drug Abuse, NIDA. For a recent review please see Vokow et al. 2016) which has shed serious light on the disorder. Via the rapidly advancing brain imaging technology particularly *functional magnetic resonance imaging (fMRI)* she and her many co-workers were able to demonstrate a deficit in the management of salient input in these patients.

Furthermore, the advancing field of medication-assisted recovery from dependence is yet more evidence that, in fact, there is something wrong with the brain mechanisms of addicted individuals. Last but of course not least is the evidence from genetic research again showing the genetic inheritance of an individual contributes towards their likelihood of developing the disorder and affects the ability to resist the temptation to fall off the wagon.

Interesting work from the field of brain event-related potentials (ERPs) adds to the understanding and perhaps may eventually be useful as a guide to treatment and rehabilitation. ERPs are measures of brain electrical activity that are induced by specific stimuli (both physical and psychological). Salvatore Campanella and his group at the Free University of Brussels (Belgium) have now shown that when a person needs to engage executive functions such as inhibition (mainly implemented in frontal lobes) harder in order to avoid the effect of a drug-related stimulus, his or her likelihood of relapsing is higher

(Campanella, 2016). If this important finding is replicated, it may have significant implications on the resources to be marshaled to help a particular individual succeed in remaining abstinent. Even more amazing is the demonstration that one of the many rapidly evolving (non-invasive) brain stimulation techniques was able to help the subjects decrease the frontal lobe effort they needed to accomplish the same task (Terraneo et al. 2016). Furthermore, cognitive training to improve inhibitory control has also shown promising results (Allom et al. 2016). The implication, which still needs to be born out via experimentation, is that individuals who are at especially high risk for relapse may find help from a variety of sources now including medications and brain stimulation technology in addition to the also proven useful peer support. In the field of substance abuse two Humanist principles are very much in evidence: the belief in science and the optimism that the human intellect can resolve any problem no matter how complicated or difficult it appears at the outset.

EDUCATION

It is the responsibility of academic centers to be the beacons of education of the societies where they exist. This is so crucial in all aspects of medicine (e.g., early warning signs of strokes or heart attacks), but is crucial for the field of psychiatry to move into the era of prevention, early detection and early effective intervention. This applies to all psychiatric disorders and equally to substance abuse. Parental education is crucial. There are well-characterized early warning signs. It is also well-known that substance use/dependence is very frequently co-morbid with other psychiatric disorders like major depression or one of the many *anxiety* disorders. Hence the early recognition of the problem allows the parents to seek advice and guidance regarding their loved ones.

Early and Effective Treatment

Here we run into a serious problem with the stigmatizing nature of psychiatric care. Many individuals will not want to be seen in psychiatric settings. This situation was contributed to by many factors, including movies, but also by the field itself. The fact that the field of psychiatry at large is seriously resistant to adopting neuroscience as the basic essential knowledge necessary for practicing helps perpetuate the stigmatizing nature of psychiatric care. In fact, the way out of stigma must pass though the BRAIN.

It is essential in this regard to actually know the facts. Would an occasional consumption of marijuana be detrimental to a person's life and career? There are two ways to answer this: via science or otherwise. The problem with the science route is that the answer takes a long time to become established and widely accepted. Implementation of scientific findings also demands resources and dedicated effort and planning.

Let's Discuss Decriminalization

For decades now we have waged a holy war on drugs. According to all the evidence we have lost. After the spectacular failure of the prohibition, the US did not learn the lesson and only recently is the recreational use of marijuana beginning to gain wide acceptance. I, in fact, never understood why equally or at times more harmful drugs like alcohol or nicotine would be legal while individuals caught with small amounts of marijuana were in jails and cluttering up an already overburdened legal system.

The answer is simple and the Humanist Principles can guide us here. Based on the science, we know these are brain disorders that remain not fully understood. Based on the "Worth and Dignity of Every Human" principle, every afflicted person must be able to receive the best care available. And only through supporting scientific research (which has already proven its worth and capabilities) will we eventually conquer this class of ailments.

Lessons from Portugal

In 2009, The CATO Institute published a report regarding the decriminalization of all drugs in Portugal (Greenwald G, 2009). This is a summary of the report.

On July 1, 2001, a nationwide law in Portugal took effect that decriminalized all drugs, including cocaine and heroin. Under the new legal framework, all drugs were "decriminalized," not "legalized." Thus, drug possession for personal use and drug usage itself were still legally prohibited, but violations of those prohibitions were deemed to be exclusively administrative violations and were removed completely from the criminal realm. Drug trafficking continued to be prosecuted as a criminal offense. While other states in the European Union have developed various forms of de facto decriminalization—whereby substances perceived to be less serious (such as cannabis) rarely lead to criminal prosecution—Portugal remains the only EU member state with a law explicitly declaring drugs to be "decriminalized." Seven years after the enactment of Portugal's decriminalization system, there were ample data that enabled its effects to be assessed. Notably, decriminalization had become increasingly popular in Portugal since 2001. Except for some far-right politicians, very few domestic political factions were agitating for a repeal of the 2001 law. And while there was a widespread perception that bureaucratic changes needed to be made to Portugal's decriminalization framework to make it more efficient and effective, there was no real debate about whether drugs should once again be criminalized.

More significantly, none of the nightmare scenarios touted by pre-enactment decriminalization opponents—from rampant increases in drug usage among the young to the transformation of Lisbon into a haven for "drug tourists"— occurred. The political consensus in favor of decriminalization is unsurprising in light of the relevant empirical data. Those data indicate that decriminalization has had no adverse effect on drug usage rates in Portugal, which, in numerous categories, are now among the lowest in the EU, particularly when compared with those with stringent criminalization regimes. Although post-decriminalization usage rates have remained roughly the same or even decreased slightly when compared with other EU states, drug-related pathologies—such as sexually transmitted diseases and deaths due to drug usage—have decreased dramatically. Drug policy experts attribute those positive trends to the enhanced ability of the Portuguese government to offer treatment programs to its citizens—enhancements made possible, for numerous reasons, by decriminalization.

In summary, the data show that, judged by virtually every metric, the Portuguese decriminalization framework has been a resounding success. Within this success lie self-evident lessons that should guide drug policy debates around the world. The question is whether the decriminalization is the optimum approach to deal with drug use and addiction or going the final step of actual legalization can have additional benefits. This issue can only be resolved via actually having the courage to try it out and learn from the results.

The Switzerland Experience

Switzerland and other countries, such as Portugal (as detailed above) and Uruguay, have implemented policies that are people-centered, focused on health and most importantly, keeping people alive. Switzerland's federal government focused on reducing the harm of drug use among people who inject drugs, creating supervised injection sites and offering substance analysis services and access to opiate substitution therapy, mainly through methadone and even medical heroin. Switzerland also complemented these harm-reduction interventions with prevention programs. To ensure these policies had citizen acceptance, the Swiss government created forums aimed at overcoming the stigma and marginalization of people who use drugs. As the Prime Minister at the time (Ruth Dreifuss) stated and reported in CNN (2016), "Our success with these policies is not only reflected in the stories that we hear from people who use drugs, but also from the rigorous evaluation we have undertaken. According to government officials, in the first decade alone, drug-related deaths have been reduced by 50%, and approximately 1,300 dependent users are now given maintenance doses of heroin via 23 specialized clinics, which has resulted in an 82% drop in patients selling heroin on the streets. We have succeeded in keeping more people alive, while respecting their human rights and increasing their access to health services."

Is it possible that it is that simple?

The answer must be highly unlikely. First, Portugal is a relatively small country and what succeeds there may not apply to much larger and perhaps more heterogeneous societies like the USA. Cerdá et al. (2011) examined medical marijuana laws in 50 states and investigated the relationship between state legalization of medical marijuana and marijuana use, abuse, and dependence. They used the second wave of the National Epidemiologic Survey on Alcohol and Related Conditions (NESARC), a national survey of adults aged 18+ (n = 34,653). Selected analyses were replicated using the National Survey on Drug Use and Health (NSDUH), a yearly survey of ~68,000 individuals aged 12+. They measured past-year cannabis use and DSM-IV abuse/dependence. In NESARC, residents of states with medical marijuana laws had higher odds of marijuana use (OR: 1.92; 95% CI: 1.49–2.47) and marijuana abuse/dependence (OR: 1.81; 95% CI: 1.22–2.67) than residents of states without such laws. Marijuana abuse/dependence was not more prevalent among marijuana users in these states (OR: 1.03; 95% CI: 0.67–1.60), suggesting that the higher risk for marijuana abuse/dependence in these states was accounted for by higher rates of use. In NSDUH, states that legalized medical marijuana also had higher rates of marijuana use. They strongly suggested that additional research needs to examine whether the association is causal, or is due to an underlying common cause, such as community norms supportive of the legalization of medical marijuana and of marijuana use.

From a humanistic view point, the bottom line is that individuals must be made to feel safe to seek help, and help must be readily and competently available.

Chapter 11

CORRECTIONAL PSYCHIATRY

INTRODUCTION

Anti-Social Personality Disorder (ASPD) is one of the most (if not the most) stigmatizing psychiatric disorders. ASPD diagnosis is usually reserved to bad actors who raise havoc on psychiatric wards, particularly in forensic psychiatry settings. It is rare, at least whenever I looked, to find the criteria by which a particular patient earned himself (and it is overwhelmingly a "he") this diagnosis. Of course, once the diagnosis is pinned on an individual, it is never questioned by the many successive psychiatrists. The ASPD diagnosis is not only stigmatizing but can also be quite harmful, given that there is no accepted effective treatment and it engenders fear from providers and caretakers, thus rendering both placement and rehabilitation challenging.

IS ASPD A BRAIN DISORDER?

What is most amazing about the disorder is that despite the harm to self that results from the behavior, patients continue to emit the same behavior. This completely defies how a normal brain works. The prefrontal regions, particularly medial prefrontal (closer to the center of the brain) and orbital prefrontal regions (just above the eyes) are equipped and designed to help us learn what is advantageous and do more of it and what is not and avoid it. Moreover, the Cingulate gyrus (a major brain track connecting many regions) is our major conflict resolution brain system. Going from anterior to posterior the level of the severity of the conflict to be resolved increases, with anterior parts more concerned with lesser conflicts (Clark et al. 2017). Furthermore, twin studies as well as other study designs have shown convincingly that there is a genetic component to the disorder (Iofrida et al. 2014). Finally, animal models for ASPD have been developed (Coccaro et al. 2011). The mere fact that many antisocial traits can be replicated in animal models points strongly to the biological bases of such traits.

Is ASPD a Homogeneous Disorder?

The answer to this question cannot be anything but no. As with all other psychiatric disorders it must be heterogeneous. Heterogeneity among psychiatric disorders is a major plague and obstacle in the face of research. Co-morbidity (also common among ASPD patients particularly for substance use and dependence) is the other major obstacle to the eventual characterization of the neurobiological mechanisms underlying such severe aberrations.

As a young neuropsychiatrist I had the fortune of being able to work patients up for organic brain involvement despite the cost attended with this work-up and the general lack of empathy from staff towards them. Among consecutive county hospitals (acute care facilities) the majority of patients with ASPD diagnosis had enough evidence of organic brain dysfunction (from mainly neuropsychology testing, CT scanning or EEG) to warrant changing the diagnosis to the then DSM-III "Organic Personality Disorder" (Hollister & Boutros, 1991; Boutros et al. 1991; Nelson & Boutros, 1993). Organic Personality Disorder is the only personality disorder that was allowed to be on Axis-I during the multiaxial diagnostic era. Organic Personality Disorder (OPD) is not a prevalent diagnosis due to the prevailing standard of work up and the reliance on historical data as well as the cost associated with an organic work-up. As such patients, while never stated so, are deemed less than worthy of such investment, it is an uphill battle to move the field of psychiatry, let alone the general, rather unsympathetic public, to invest heavily in this population. This is particularly sad as major advances have been made in both cognitive remediation (Kaldoja et al. 2015) and in the understanding of how the inhibitory/excitatory neurotransmitter balances occur in the brain. Cognitive remediation/retraining is based on the accumulating knowledge regarding brain plasticity. It is well known that plasticity (i.e., the ability of the brain to change its structure) is better the younger the age. As the majority of ASPD diagnoses are given to relatively young individuals (at times even in their teens) this fact thus represents a major hope that if the correct diagnosis is made (i.e., organic personality disorder vs. ASPD) the more likely the patient can be rehabilitated via cognitive retraining. Even more promising is the ever-advancing capability of administering the retraining via computers thus decreasing the cost of treatment. Cognitive retraining, simply defined, depends on identification of the cognitive deficits in an individual, designing cognitive retraining programs (which tends to look like computer games), administering the training and following up with cognitive testing to monitor and assess progress.

Early Psychiatric Testing Is Imperative in Changing the Trajectory of the Disorder

It is well-documented, in fact required by the DSM diagnostic system, that the individual being evaluated for an ASPD diagnosis must have exhibited aberrant behavior (e.g., conduct disorder) before the age of 15. This occurs years or even decades before an individual commits an act that earns him either jail (or at times much worse), or long-term (and rather expensive) hospitalization. A full medical and neurological work up (including a full battery of neuropsychological testing) at this junction must not be denied to these individuals and their families. Similarly, a full psychosocial assessment must be rendered to identify if any modifiable factors are perpetuating the behavior. Close follow-up and management of these young individuals should not be optional and well-designed and well-funded programs need to be developed.

Psychiatrists and Psychologists Must Never Be Wardens

During the late stages of my career, I worked in a setting where I was, in fact, a warden. I had the most harming patient-doctor relationship. I was responsible for forcing patients to take medications against their will (including tying them down and administering injectable medications). This went against everything I believed in and wanted to do as a physician.

HOSPITALS MUST NOT BE JAILS and judges should NEVER be allowed to force patients into hospitals.

It is quite possible to build hospitals inside correctional systems. Psychiatrists can provide the clinical care to incarcerated patients but must never themselves be the jailers. This allows for a more therapeutic relationship to develop. Patient cooperation with treatment recommendation can be figured into the nature and duration of the sentence.

The dilemma of "competency restoration" to stand trial must also be closely examined. It is well-known that one of the most crucial factors for recovery is the development of insight. By forcing patients into treatment, we can get some improvement, but what is the evidence for long-term effectiveness? If the sole purpose is to allow a patient to be tried, this also needs to be done in a jail setting where a patient may be more motivated to want to be released.

COMPETENCY TO STAND TRIAL

In 2013 there were 91,266 criminal cases filed in court in the United States. In order for all of those 91,266 cases to be heard in 2013, the criminal defendant had to be judged legally competent to stand trial. Due process requires that a defendant be competent to stand trial. Trying a person who is not competent is said to offend the dignity of the court, to undermine the credibility of the State, and to deprive the citizen of essential rights. The competence examination of a defendant is guided by the conclusions in the case, Dusky v. United States, 271 F.2d 385, 395 (8th Cir. Mo. 1959), which set down the two cardinal elements of competency to stand trial. First, the defendant must have a rational as well as factual understanding of the charges against him or her and the penalties associated with them. Second, the defendant must have the ability to cooperate with an attorney in his or her own defense (US Legal Inc, 1997). If a criminal defendant is named to be Incompetent to Stand Trial (IST), the defendant is forced to receive treatment resulting from the IST trial of Sell V. U.S where a person named to be IST was sentenced with mandated hospitalization in hopes it would restore the defendant's competency. While hospitalized the defendant refused medication, and to force administration of the medication the magistrate claimed that Sell was a danger to himself and others. The magistrate was forcing restoration of competency so the defendant could stand trial and receive judgment to possibly be incarcerated. The state of California spent approximately $170 million annually on significant resources to provide treatment for this population, which in 2012 was between 200 and 300 IST patients. The prison environment enables the worsening of preexisting mental disabilities thus completely undoing all previous restoration and hospital efforts. After incarceration, defendants will most likely be incarcerated again thus being stuck in this cyclical legal process.

We here question the efficacy and humanity of restoring a criminal defendant to competency in order to stand trial and then sending him/her to a very stressful situation like incarceration. We believe that incarceration following restoration is likely to undo that initial restoration or even be a further detriment to the competence of the defendant.

The most common psychiatric conditions of IST patients are medication resistant schizophrenia, delusional disorder (DD), Bipolar disorder (BD), organic cognitive disorder, including impulse dyscontrol and sexual predation and violence as well as antisocial and borderline personality disorders. Some of the most common psychiatric disorders that are mistreated or ignored in prisons are phobic anxiety disorders (agoraphobia, social phobia and specific phobias), other anxiety disorders (panic disorder and generalized anxiety disorder), and dissociative (conversion) disorders (RSMO, 2016). These disorders need psychotherapy which is highly unlikely to be available in a jail setting.

Jails and prisons are required to provide basic health care for inmates, but the quality of this care varies greatly. Often, prison-based mental health care focuses on stabilizing, rather than treating inmates, thus completely undoing all previous restoration and hospital efforts to treat them. By providing inferior and inadequate health care for defendants, the system is violating their right to health and their right to Humane Treatment and Rehabilitation.

Article 10(1) of the International Covenant on Civil and Political Rights (ICCPR), to which the United States is a party, expressly requires all prisoners to be treated, by all officials and anyone else, "with humanity and with respect for the inherent dignity of the human person."

CORRECTIONAL MENTAL HEALTH CARE

According to the Human Rights Watch, the United States is a signatory to the right to health, and is thus bound to honoring its responsibilities - that states must ensure "the right of everyone to the enjoyment of the highest attainable standard of physical and mental health." It is stated that "while the state validly exercises a restraint on those persons who are a detriment to its public social order, there exists a corresponding duty to those persons detained to give them care, cure, and treatment (Bassiouni 1966). To insure this right, states must create "conditions which would assure all medical services and medical attention in the event of sickness."

The Committee on Economic, Social and Cultural Rights (ICESCR) interprets the right to health under article 12 of the ICESCR places states "under the obligation to respect the right to health by, inter alia, refraining from denying or limiting equal access for all persons, including prisoners or detainees, to preventive, curative and palliative health services" (Bassiouni 1966). However, prisons have found this particularly hard as a result of the increasing number of inmates who require mental health care. Paula M. Ditton, a statistician at the Bureau of Justice Statistics (BJS), reported that at midyear 1998, an estimated 283,800 mentally ill offenders were incarcerated in the nation's prisons and jails. "In a 2006 Special Report, the BJS estimated that 705,600 mentally ill adults were incarcerated in state prisons, 78,800 in federal prisons and 479,900 in local jails (Prins, Jacob, and Draper, 2009)." Not having access to proper health care is a major detriment to a person susceptible to competency de-restoration. As prisons and jails continue to become more and more over capacity, the level of health care will continue to decrease due to lack of recourses, including adequate staffing and funding.

Sending IST patients to prison and having them enter the mental health conditions in correctional facilities violates the defendant's right to Humane Treatment and Rehabilitation. The Human Rights Watch has affirmed that the application of article 10, promoting the right to humane treatment, "cannot be dependent on the material resources available."

Principle 9 of the UN ""Basic Principles for the Treatment of Prisoners" states, "Prisoners shall have access to the health services available in the country without discrimination on the grounds of their legal situation." Similarly, principle 20 of the UN Principles for the Protection of Persons with Mental Illnesses and the Improvement of Mental Health Care states that all persons serving sentences "should receive the best available mental health care" with treatment and care consistent with that outlined for individuals who are not incarcerated.

However, this right to health is violated as seen through cases of the previously stated disorders: Phobic anxiety disorders (agoraphobia, social phobia and specific phobias), other anxiety disorders (panic disorder and generalized anxiety disorder), and dissociative [conversion] disorders]. The previously mentioned BJS report by Paula M. Ditton in July 1999 reported the percentages of inmates who needed a certain level of mental health care during incarceration in a federal prison: 45.6% received counseling or therapy, and 49.1 had taken a prescribed medication. A person experiencing hallucinations or psychosis might get medication to control the most severe symptoms, but people with anxiety issues, depression, post-traumatic stress, and other mental health conditions that don't cause radical changes in behavior may go untreated. These latter conditions are recognized to be associated with significant suicidality and co-morbidity with other disorders, including substance dependence. Contrary to the common belief these conditions are not less serious than the psychotic disorders. Prisoners rarely, if ever, get therapy or comprehensive treatment, so mental health issues that were previously controlled with medication and therapy may get much worse during incarceration.

Isolation

Correctional facilities create an environment of isolation through their limited access to the outside world, thus increasing the difficulty of reentering society. Many jails have instituted mail policies prohibiting letters and magazine subscriptions, and these policies can eliminate prisoners' ability to stay connected to the outside world as well as communicate with and receive support from loved ones. Isolation can increase a person's risk of mental health issues such as depression and anxiety. This level of isolation increases with the decreased support they have on the outside.

It is well known that the new generations of psychotropic medications are significantly more expensive than the older psychotropic medications. It is logical that many agencies, particularly correctional agencies, do not have enough funds to support all the patients in their custody who are in need of such medications. Many states, in the enactment of mental health codes or statutes, refer to persons in need of cure and treatment. It is not stretching the rules of interpretation too far to conclude that if the statute is applicable to a person who is in need of mental treatment, that individual is entitled to receive that cure and treatment" (Bassiouni 1966). This problem also affects the clinical decision-making of the providers working on restoring the patient's mental health. For example, clinicians may restrict their choice of medications to the medications that the patient is likely to be able to receive in the correctional facility.

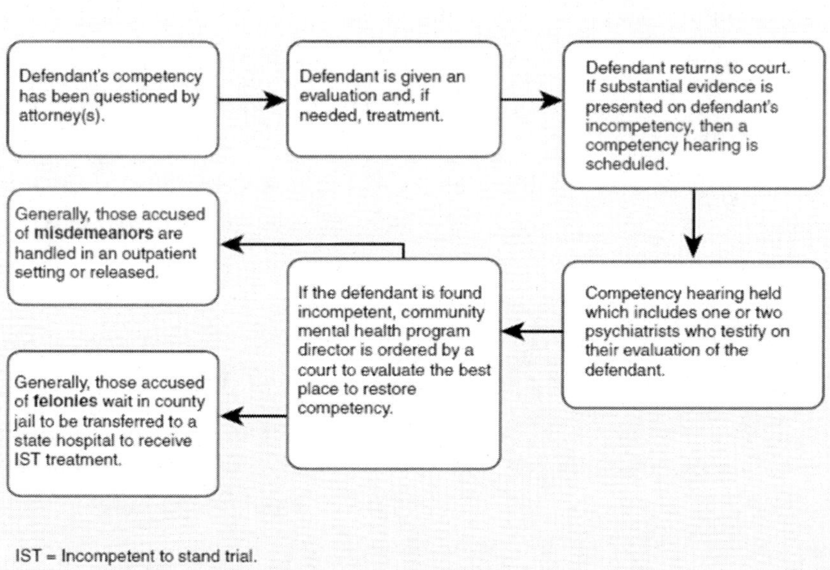

Figure 2. Step-wise progression of the process by which a defendant is found to be incompetent to stand trial (IST) and placed in a state facility.

The Cyclical Problem of "Recidivism"

That is what makes this process cyclical. If the restoration of the defendant's competency is undone due to factors involving the prison system, the likelihood of their committing an offense again is just as high, if not higher than when they committed the first crime. If the defendant is judged incompetent to stand trial again, he will have to go through the entire restoration process again, which includes both the medical restorations and the legal IST commitment process. This IST commitment process is laid out in Figure 2.

Conclusion

The environment in prisons due to the violation of the right to health and the right to treatment and rehabilitation, leads to the worsening of mental disabilities and the probability of re-committing a criminal act followed by reincarceration. The volatile and expensive outcome is that the number of IST patients stuck in this never-ending prison loop exponentially increases at a very fast rate; the old IST patients never leave the prison cycle and new IST patients enter.

Inmates incarcerated for violent crimes do not typically serve life sentences. Most prisoners are ultimately released, and the mental health issues they developed in prison can increase their risk of reoffending and make it difficult to reenter society as productive, non-threatening citizens. Almost 70% of people who have been incarcerated are arrested again within three years, and the dire state of mental health care in prisons plays a significant role in perpetuating this high rate of recidivism.

There is a lot of controversy regarding the incarceration of previously IST patients. Some believe these people are still criminals. Yes, they got treatment, but they still committed a crime, and it is believed that any person who commits a crime should be held accountable and punished. In contrast, it is believed by Professor Randy Otto, that "Trying those who are so impaired that they cannot aid in their defense or are unaware of the nature and purpose of the proceedings against them is considered to challenge both the dignity of the legal process and conceptions about fundamental fairness" (Otto 2006).

When individuals who committed offenses are judged to be IST they can be managed in two fundamentally different ways. They can be entered into the above restoration-incarceration-release-reoffending cycle, which is most common, or they can be released to the community with close monitoring while receiving psychiatric care. Whether one of these two routes is superior to the other is a serious question. Based on a thorough review of available research (which remains limited) we were able to conclude that the release into the community with close supervision is superior for the short term with regards to re-offending. We were also able to conclude that there are no long-term prospective randomized studies designed to compare the clinical and legal outcome of restored individuals with similar levels of psychiatric problems and similar degrees of offenses when randomized to incarceration and usual correctional psychiatric care vs. rehabilitation in the community with close psychiatric care. Without such prospectively well-designed studies the above questions may remain unanswered (Boutros et al. 2018).

We here strongly advocate a very close collaboration between academic institutions and the correctional system. The nature of patients in the system does not easily lend itself to the sort of research that the NIH or NSF would support. By staffing state hospitals with the highest caliber physicians and psychologists, the field could, in fact, advance.

Chapter 12

Developmental Intellectual Disabilities: Formerly Mental Retardation

Introduction

As of the writing of this book the fields of preventing, diagnosing, and managing developmental intellectual disabilities are not integrated into the larger field of Psychiatry. The majority of adult psychiatrists receive no exposure to this area of knowledge and do not develop any expertise in dealing with this difficult patient population. Child psychiatrists do get some exposure to this area but as is well known, all the patients become adults and continue to need help. Again, as of the writing of this book, there are very few specialized training programs to help clinicians who find themselves having to care for these patients. The good news is that a movement is underway to increase the number of such advanced fellowship training programs in the US.

Developmental Intellectual Disability (DID) is by definition a permanent condition that results from an insult or a genetically determined defect to the developing brain. Such disabilities again by definition deprive the individuals from having a full functioning cognitive capacity before they even start life.

The goal for all efforts must be the eventual elimination of DID in all its forms. Humanity was successful in all but eliminating polio and small pox, and this is as worthy a goal as eliminating these other ailments.

There are at least three phases for possible intervention:

1. Preconception genetic counseling. A growing body of knowledge is unraveling the many genetic and epigenetic causes for intellectual disabilities. This will allow potential parents to make informed decisions. As attested to by a growing literature, many pre-conception factors are modifiable including stress, substance abuse, and malnutrition.
2. When parents decide to take their chances following genetic counseling, they can also decide to closely monitor the development of the fetus. Modern day technology allows the detection of deviations within days of conception. This is available to all parents and as technology improves, the cost of testing should progressively come down. The implication here is clear. When testing indicates a certain degree of damage (that is deemed unacceptable by the society norms at the time) then the pregnancy is terminated. Even in the face of most restrictive abortion laws (similar to what is being proposed for Texas during the writing of this book), this technology will be very useful as it can be informative well before the six-weeks limit being proposed in Texas.
3. The third phase for intervention occurs too late and should be a last resort. That is to mitigate the damage that has already occurred via immediate and full-blown intervention. (Cost should NEVER come into the equation.) A full assessment of the newborn with close follow up should allow early intervention. All possible resources should be marshaled to help the child grow as healthy and be as integrated as possible.

RECENT RESEARCH EFFORTS TOWARDS THE ABOVE GOALS

A good example is a book edited by Howson CP, Kennedy ET, Horwitz A, *Prevention of Micronutrient Deficiencies: Tools for Policymakers and Public Health Workers*, 1998. This volume combines some but not all of the above approaches. Micronutrient malnutrition affects approximately 2 billion people worldwide. The adverse effects of micronutrient deficiencies are profound and include premature death, poor health, blindness, growth stunting, mental retardation, learning disabilities, and low work capacity. *Prevention of Micronutrient Deficiencies* provides a conceptual framework based on past experience that will allow funders to tailor programs to existing regional/country capabilities and to incorporate within these programs the capacity to address multiple strategies (i.e., supplementation/fortification/food-based approaches/public health measures) and multiple micronutrient deficiencies. The book does not offer recommendations on how to alleviate specific micronutrient deficiencies. Such recommendations are already available through the publications of diverse organizations, including the U.S. Agency for International Development, the Micronutrient Initiative, World Bank, United Nations Children's Fund, and the World Health Organization. Instead, this volume examines key elements in the design and implementation of micronutrient interventions, including such issues as the importance of iron, vitamin A, and iodine to health. Populations at risk for micronutrient deficiency are identified and options for successful interventions and their costs are highlighted.

A report by Brites & Fernandes highlights the existence of critical time windows that may be crucial to institute intervention (Brites & Fernandes, 2015). Bilirubin-induced neurologic dysfunction (BIND) and classical kernicterus are clinical manifestations of moderate to severe hyperbilirubinemia whenever bilirubin levels exceed the capacity of the brain's defensive mechanisms in preventing its entrance and cytotoxicity.

In such circumstances and depending on the associated co-morbidities, bilirubin accumulation may lead to short- or long-term neurodevelopmental disabilities, which may include deficits in auditory, cognitive, and motor processing.

Van Karnebeek & Stockler (2012) reviewed the causes of treatable inborn errors of metabolism causing intellectual disability. They defined intellectual disability as developmental delay at age<5 years and reported that 2.5% of population worldwide is affected. Recommendations to investigate genetic causes of intellectual disability are based on frequencies of single conditions and on the yield of diagnostic methods, rather than the availability of causal therapy. Inborn errors of metabolism constitute a subgroup of rare genetic conditions for which an increasing number of treatments has become available. They assessed levels of evidence of treatments and characterized the effect of treatments on IQ/development and related outcomes. They identified a total of 81 "treatable inborn errors of metabolism" presenting with intellectual disability as a major feature. Sixty-two % of all disorders are identified by metabolic screening tests in the blood (plasma amino acids, homocysteine) and urine (creatine metabolites, glycosaminoglycans, oligosaccharides, organic acids, pyrimidines). For the remaining disorders a "single test per single disease" approach, including primary molecular analysis, is required. Therapeutic modalities include: sick-day management, diet, co-factor/vitamin supplements, substrate inhibition, stem cell transplant, and gene therapy. Therapeutic effects include improvement and/or stabilization of psychomotor/cognitive development, behavior/psychiatric disturbances, seizures, and neurologic and systemic manifestations. They then concluded that this literature review generated the evidence to prioritize treatability in the diagnostic evaluation of intellectual disability. The results were translated into digital information tools for the clinician (www.treatable-id.org), which are part of a diagnostic protocol, currently implemented for an evaluation of the effectiveness in their institution. Treatments for these disorders are relatively accessible, affordable, and with acceptable side-effects. Evidence for the majority of the therapies is limited however.

International collaborations, patient registries, and novel trial methodologies are key to turning the tide for rare diseases such as these.

In a similar vein, Grosse & Van Vliet (2011) examined the possibility of the prevention of intellectual disability through screening for congenital hypothyroidism. They stated that congenital hypothyroidism (CHT) is a common cause of preventable mental retardation, and the quantification of intellectual disability due to CHT is needed to assess the public health benefit of newborn screening. Towards this end, they reviewed published studies conducted among children born prior to the introduction of newborn screening for CHT and reported cognitive test scores. Their study included children with clinically diagnosed CHT and instituted thyroid hormone substitution and examined Intelligence quotient (IQ) (mean and distribution) as their main outcome measure. They reported that the prevalence of recognized CHT rose from one in 6500 prior to screening to approximately one in 3000 with screening. In four population-based studies in high-income countries, among children with clinically diagnosed CHT 8-28% were classified as having intellectual disability (defined as an IQ < 70) and the mean IQ was 85 (a leftward shift of 1 SD). Among children with subclinical CHT, the risk of overt intellectual disability was lower (zero in one study), but decreased intellectual potential and increased behavioral abnormalities were documented. They concluded that although the prevalence of overt disability among children with CHT in the absence of screening may be less than previously estimated, the preventable burden of intellectual disability due to CHT is substantial and justifies newborn screening. However, changes in existing newborn screening protocols to capture more cases are unlikely to prevent overt cases of disability and should therefore be justified instead by the documentation of other benefits of early detection.

More recently, Ford & LaFranchi (2014) further addressed the screening for congenital hypothyroidism. They agreed that detection by newborn screening (NBS) and treatment of babies with congenital hypothyroidism (CH) has largely eliminated the intellectual disability caused by this disorder. Lowering of the screening TSH cutoff and changes in birth demographics have been associated with an approximate doubling of the incidence of CH, from 1:3500 to 1:1714. The additional cases detected by lowering of the TSH cutoff tend to have milder hypothyroidism. Imaging, in these cases, often demonstrated a eutopic, "gland in-situ," and some cases turn out to have transient CH. Based on their search for the then current screening programs, approximately 71 percent of babies worldwide are not born in an area with an established NBS program, despite the existence of screening for over five decades in developed countries. Thus, the majority of babies with CH worldwide are not detected and treated early. As a result, the economic burden of retardation owing to CH remains a significant public health challenge.

Skeaff (2011) probed the effect on neurodevelopment in the child of Iodine deficiency in pregnancy which is another readily preventable factor. Iodine is an integral part of the thyroid hormones, thyroxine (T4) and tri-iodothyronine (T(3)), necessary for normal growth and development. An adequate supply of cerebral T(3), generated in the fetal brain from maternal free T4 (fT4), is needed by the fetus for thyroid hormone dependent neurodevelopment, which begins in the second half of the first trimester of pregnancy. Around the beginning of the second trimester, the fetal thyroid also begins to produce hormones but the reserves of the fetal gland are low. Thus maternal thyroid hormones contribute to total fetal thyroid hormone concentrations until birth. In order for pregnant women to produce enough thyroid hormones to meet both their own and their baby's requirements, a 50% increase in iodine intake is recommended. A lack of iodine in the diet may result in the mother becoming iodine deficient, and subsequently the fetus. In iodine deficiency, hypothyroxinemia (i.e., low maternal fT(4)) results in damage to the developing brain, which is further aggravated by hypothyroidism in the fetus. The most serious consequence of iodine deficiency is cretinism, characterized by profound mental retardation. There is unequivocal evidence that severe iodine deficiency in pregnancy impairs brain development in the child. However, only two intervention trials have assessed neurodevelopment in the children of moderately iodine deficient mothers, finding improved neurodevelopment in children of mothers supplemented earlier rather than later in pregnancy. Both studies were not randomized and were uncontrolled. Thus, there is a need for well-designed trials to determine the effect of iodine supplementation in moderate to mildly iodine deficient pregnant women on the neurodevelopment in the child.

Additional societal risk factors that can be addressed were highlighted by Lambert et al. (2013). High-risk environments characterized by familial substance use, poverty, inadequate parental monitoring, and exposure to violence are associated with an increased propensity for adolescents to engage in risk-taking behaviors (e.g., substance use, sexual behavior, and delinquency). However, additional factors, such as drug exposure in-utero and deficits in inhibitory control among drug-exposed youth, may further influence the likelihood that adolescents in high-risk environments will engage in risk-taking behavior. This study examined the influence of prenatal substance exposure, inhibitory control, and sociodemographic/environmental risk factors on risk-taking behaviors in a large cohort of adolescents with and without prenatal cocaine exposure (PCE). Risk-taking behavior (delinquency, substance use, and sexual activity) was assessed in 963 adolescents (433 cocaine-exposed, 530 non-exposed) at 15 years of age. Prenatal cocaine exposure predicted later arrests and early onset of sexual behavior in controlled analyses. In addition, male gender, low parental involvement, and exposure to violence were associated with greater odds of engaging in risk-taking behavior across the observed domains. The authors concluded that the study findings substantiate concern regarding the association between prenatal substance exposure and related risk factors and the long-term outcomes of exposed youth. Access to the appropriate social, educational, and medical services is essential in preventing and intervening with risk-taking behaviors and their potential consequences (e.g., adverse health outcomes and incarceration), especially among high-risk adolescent youths and their families.

The genetics of early onset cognitive impairment have been less well-examined (Ropers, 2012). DID is the leading socio-economic problem of health care, but compared to autism and schizophrenia, it has received very little public attention. Important risk factors for ID are malnutrition, cultural deprivation, poor health care, and parental consanguinity (marriages among relatives). In the Western world, fetal alcohol exposure is the most common preventable cause. Most severe forms of ID have genetic causes. Cytogenetically detectable (sophisticated method to examine cell structure) and submicroscopic chromosomal rearrangements account for approximately 25% of all cases. X-linked gene defects are responsible in 10-12% of males with ID. To date, 91 of these defects have been identified. In contrast, autosomal gene defects have been largely disregarded, but due to coordinated efforts and the advent of next-generation DNA sequencing, this is about to change. As shown for Fra(X) syndrome, this renewed focus on autosomal gene defects will pave the way for molecular diagnosis and prevention, shed more light on the pathogenesis (i.e., how a disease develops) of ID, and reveal new opportunities for therapy.

Franklin & Mansuy (2011) addressed the involvement of epigenetic (i.e., effects of environmental factors on genetics) defects in mental retardation. They asserted that while the diseases associated with mental retardation are diverse, a significant number are linked with disruptions in epigenetic mechanisms, mainly due to loss-of-function mutations in genes that are key components of the epigenetic machinery. Additionally, several disorders classed as imprinting syndromes are associated with mental retardation. Musante & Ropers (2014) examined the genetics of recessive cognitive disorders and reported that most severe forms of intellectual disability (ID) have specific genetic causes. Numerous X chromosome gene defects and disease-causing copy-number variants have been linked to ID and related disorders, and recent studies have revealed that sporadic cases are often due to dominant de novo mutations with low recurrence risk. For autosomal recessive ID (ARID) the recurrence risk is high and, in populations with frequent parental consanguinity, ARID is the most common form of ID. Even so, its elucidation has lagged behind.

Prenatal *substance use* is a major public health problem and a social morbidity, with consequences on the drug user and the offspring.

Sithisarn, et al. (2012) reported on the consequences of prenatal substance use. Their review focused on the child and adolescent outcomes following in-utero drug exposure. Studies on the effects of specific substances, legal and illegal; i.e., tobacco or nicotine, alcohol, marijuana, cocaine, opiates, and methamphetamines were evaluated and analyzed. In general, they found that manifestations of prenatal exposure to legal and illegal substances include varying deficits in birth anthropometric (normal ranges of height and weight) measurements, mild-to-moderate transient neurobehavioral alterations in infancy and long-term behavioral problems noted from early childhood to adolescence. The severity of the expression of behavioral problems is influenced by environmental factors. Further, behavioral alterations following in utero drug exposure often exist with psychiatric co-morbidities. They concluded that because of the long-term consequences of prenatal drug exposure on child and adolescent mental health, health providers need to promote substance use prevention, screen for exposure effects and provide or refer affected youths for intervention services. Preventive measures and treatment should consider other factors that may further increase the risk of psychopathology in the exposed children.

In the 2022 world, it is hard to imagine malnutrition being a factor. Groce and collaborators (2014) investigated the relationship between malnutrition and disability. They indicated that there is increasing international interest in the links between malnutrition and disability: both are major global public health problems, both are key human rights concerns, and both are currently prominent within the global health agenda. In this review, interactions between the two fields are explored and it is argued that strengthening those links would lead to important mutual benefits and synergies. At numerous points throughout the life cycle, malnutrition can cause or contribute to an individual's physical, sensory, intellectual, or mental health disability. By working more closely together, these problems can be transformed into opportunities. Nutrition services and programs for children and adults can act as entry points to address and, in some cases, avoid or mitigate disability. Disability programs can improve nutrition for the children and adults they serve. For this to happen, however, political commitment and resources are needed, as are better data.

Mason et al. (2014) outlined "A Promise Renewed Target for Children and the Vision of Every Woman, Every Child," to focus political attention and improve performance goals for newborn babies. The "Every Newborn Series" shows the potential for a triple return on investment around the time of birth. Beyond survival, being counted and optimum nutrition and development is a human right for all children, including those with disabilities. Improved human capital brings economic productivity. Efforts to reach every woman and every newborn baby, close gaps in coverage, and improve equity and quality for antenatal, intrapartum, and postnatal care, especially in the poorest countries and for underserved populations, need urgent attention. The authors prioritized what needs to be done differently on the basis of learning from the past decade about what has worked, and what has not. Needed now are four most important shifts: (1) intensification of political attention and leadership; (2) promotion of parent voices, supporting women, families, and communities to speak up for their newborn babies and to challenge social norms that accept these disabilities as inevitable; (3) investment for changes on morbidity outcome as well as a harmonization of funding; (4) implementation at scale, with particular attention to increasing of health worker numbers and skills with attention to high-quality childbirth care for newborn babies as well as mothers and children; and (5) evaluation: tracking coverage of priority interventions and packages of care with clear accountability to accelerate progress and reach the poorest groups. The Every Newborn Action Plan provides an *evidence-based* roadmap towards care for every woman, and a healthy start for every newborn baby, with a right to be counted, survive, and thrive wherever they are born.

The Iceland Experiment and the Near Elimination of Down's Syndrome

The country of Iceland instituted a program for prenatal testing for Down's syndrome (BBC Documentary, 2016). Prenatal testing remained optional for expecting parents, but the government mandated that doctors notify women/parents of this option. Reports indicate that about 85% of informed, expectant mothers do opt for the testing. Even more importantly, close to 100% of Icelandic women chose to abort if the fetus had the possibility of Down's syndrome. It is also reported that due to faulty testing as little as two children were born in Iceland with the syndrome each year (Wise, 2016). It seems that false negative testing (a negative test despite the presence of the syndrome) usually reflects a lower level of severity of the syndrome. I was unable to find reports of false positives. In other words NO healthy fetus was aborted secondary to a wrong test. Iceland, in fact, was one of the first countries that sponsored and supported widespread pre-natal testing. Similar reports from other western European countries have emerged placing the percentile of pregnant women with positive pre-natal tests for Down's Syndrome who chose to abort at 90%. An overall rate of such decision in Europe is about 92%. Amazingly, this percentile drops to somewhere between 70 and 90% in the US.

It should be noted that a cardinal medical concept is that prevention outweighs treatment. The fact that prevention, in this case, entails an emotional and culturally difficult issue like abortion does not in any way negate the fact that prevention is superior to treatment no matter how effective the treatment may be. This Icelandic, and its European extension, highlight two very important Humanistic Principles. First is the right of humans for informed choice (Nursing Standard, 2016). Second is the Worth and Dignity of every human. In this case the parents decide that their children deserve a full chance on life and do not dictate a life with less than a full capacity for their children. Taking advantage of scientific advances is also a cornerstone of Humanism.

Boudreaux & Thompson (2015) argue both sides (for and against) the rights of the pregnant mother when it comes to substance abuse during the pregnancy. The effects of alcohol use during gestation are well-characterized. The fetal alcohol syndrome has been extensively studied but the effects of other drugs of abuse not nearly as much. They concluded that the bulk of the argument supports the need to intervene on behalf of the fetus when the mother's behavior is clearly endangering its well-being. Again, significantly more research is needed to know exactly when to intervene and how to intervene when a pregnant mother is abusing substances.

Conclusion

It is inescapable at the current time and with the knowledge that is already available that many causes of developmental intellectual disabilities can be significantly ameliorated if not eliminated altogether. It is well-documented that children and adults with developmental disabilities are at heightened risk for abuse with all its forms including sexual abuse. Despite the development of community programs to prevent such abuse it remains a very difficult problem as the developmentally disabled individual has decreased ability to self-protect as well as to seek help to stop the abuse (Harden et al. 2016). It is also clear that much more research remains necessary to completely eradicate all causes of this life-long society-burdening problem.

Chapter 13

Stigma

The issue of stigma is well known. Two main factors tend to be the major contributors to a disorder or a condition being stigmatizing. The first is attributing the problem to a personal characteristic that the person at some level is in control of, much like in sexually transmitted diseases. This is perhaps the major factor in the stigma associated with psychiatric disorders. A second factor is the uncertainty regarding what the condition could lead to. The perception that the disorder is indicative of a character flaw leads to a reluctance to hire the person. The possibility of violence or the simple fear of lack of reliability could hinder an employer from offering a job to an otherwise qualified person.

Efforts to deal with and combat the stigma associated with receiving a psychiatric diagnosis, or even just seeing a psychiatrist, are many but have had hardly any progress. The RECALCITRANT nature of the "mental" illness stigma will remain as long as the term "mental" remains. These disorders are stigmatizing because they are "mental" as opposed to regular physical disorders. As was repeatedly argued throughout this volume, our way out of stigma must go through the BRAIN. Throughout an article entitled "Fighting the stigma caused by mental disorders: past perspectives, present activities, and future directions," there was no mention of the brain, psychiatric disorders as brain disorders or neuroscience in general (Stuart, 2008). This is hardly the case now. The term "mental" embodies the duality mind-brain or mental-physical. Doing away with this duality is our first step to bury stigma and relegate it to the history of medicine.

As, most recently summarized by Gronholm et al in 2017, there is evidence that mass media campaigns and interventions for target groups had small to moderate positive impact in terms of *stigma*-related knowledge, attitudes, and intended behavior in terms of desire for contact. However, the limited evidence from longer follow-ups suggests that it is not clear whether these short-term contact interventions have a lasting impact.

The problem of stigma is even more complicated when it comes to children. Eaton and colleagues (2017) provided data from interviews with 11 mothers of children (aged 5-13 years) with mental health disorders. Mothers selectively disclosed (and concealed) to protect and advocate for their children. Their decisions were often influenced by, or were a reaction to, others' opinions, with mothers not only avoiding, but also defending against stigma, and exercising their right to privacy. They pointed to the fact that despite anticipating negative feedback, mothers more often experienced empathy and support following disclosure. They recommended that mothers' confidence in disclosing should be supported and developed. While reaching out to mothers of potentially ill children is complex, it is indeed an important step for early detection and intervention in most psychiatric disorders. The most direct way to accomplish this rather important goal is through mass education via mass media but also in kindergartens, preschools and even grade schools.

If we recall, for as long as its brain etiology, its biological cause, was unknown, "epilepsy" was a highly stigmatizing disorder. Suspected causes ranged from demonic possession to excessive masturbation. This is hardly the case now. Once the "biological" nature was fully and unequivocally identified, the disorder began to progressively lose its stigma. The stigma associated with epilepsy did not dissipate overnight and some level of stigma remains today. There is no reason to believe that the stigma associated with any psychiatric disorder will have a different fate. The stigma associated with tertiary neuro-syphilis- (general paresis of the insane or GPI) also did not dissipate except with the actual, almost, eradication of the disease itself, and that is likely because of its "morality" implications.

I would like to share a case history to illustrate a VERY important point. A sixty-year-old senior executive in a multimillion-dollar company began to slip deadlines and show up late to work, sometimes not well-kempt in appearance. His concerned wife was able to get him to see his family physician who performed a comprehensive evaluation that proved to be entirely negative. When the physician suggested that this might be "depression" and that the patient should consult with a psychiatrist, the patient became enraged at what he perceived as an incompetent physician. The concerned physician, not knowing where to turn for help, called the neurology department in the local medical school. It so happened that the department had a "neuro-psychiatry" program administered by a double-trained psychiatrist-neurologist. The clinic, which was housed in the neurology suite, allowed the patient to be seen without resentment or anger. The patient received a full neurological examination and full cognitive assessment. While the neurological exam was perfectly normal, the cognitive assessment revealed a slowing of cognition. The impression was that the patient was most likely suffering from a major depressive disorder. Knowing the history of this particular patient, the neuro-psychiatrist did not mention the diagnosis but ordered a polysomnogam (overnight sleep study) hoping that it would reveal the rapid-eye movement (REM) changes commonly associated with the condition (Arfken et al. 2014). In fact, the study revealed just that. The hypnogram summarized the results of the study, showing the sleep architecture of one whole night. During the next visit, the neuro-psychiatrist showed the patient, who was indeed very anxious to see the test results, a normal hypnogram revealing the normal 4-5 cycles with REM onset about 90 minutes from sleep onset. Once the patient's hypnogram was displayed in front of him, before any explanation was offered, the patient immediately noticed that it was very different with much fragmentation and very early REM sleep onset. The anxious patient asked about what caused that, and the answer was major depressive disorder. The surprised patient asked how a "psychological problem" could cause what was obviously a brain change.

Now the neuro-psychiatrist was able to explain the current neurotransmitter theories and the way to correct the chemical abnormality. Suffice it to say that three weeks of fluoxetine (a widely prescribed antidepressant) were sufficient for the patient to recover and be back at work.

The full recognition of the biological nature of an illness will usher in the beginning of the dissipation of the stigma.

ADVOCACY FOR PSYCHIATRICALLY ILL INDIVIDUALS

Advocacy for psychiatric patients, particularly those with severe and persistent illnesses, is weak at best and frequently completely absent. This is an astonishing fact given that one out of every five humans suffer from psychiatric disorders of one form or another. It follows that it is almost impossible to live a life with never being exposed to psychiatric disorders in a friend or a relative who is suffering. An effective organization representing this huge percentage of people could have an immense lobbying power that would assure adequate and innovative care, legal protection of individuals incarcerated due to psychiatric disorders and enough funding for research.

Currently one main organization advocates for "the mentally ill" in the US; the National Alliance for the Mentally Ill (NAMI). A number of smaller organizations do as well. The World Health Organization advocates internationally and plays a bigger role in developing countries. Smaller organizations are focused on certain types of illnesses like *schizophrenia*, bipolar disorder, etc.

Advocating for the mentally ill is a huge undertaking as approximately 20% of society suffers from one form of it or the other. One major problem with advocacy is the issue of conflict of interest. For example, when the American Psychiatric Association advocates for psychiatric care, it is by definition supporting its membership. Independent mental health advocates can play a major role (Fleischman, 2015). An independent mental health advocate (IMHA) can offer individuals detained against their will impartial support and advice. Having access to an IMHA can help patients and service users regain control of their care.

Mental health advocacy must extend to individuals with substance use disorders, particularly because for treatment to be effective, it tends to be expensive, leaving many who are either uncovered or under-covered with less than adequate management (Degenhardt, et al. 2017). Advocacy must also extend to sexual minorities (Willging et al. 2017) as well as the intellectually cognitively disabled.

The term "Mental" embodies the duality mind-brain or mental-physical. Doing away with this duality is our first step to burying stigma and relegating it to the history of medicine.

CONCLUSION

I am repeatedly asked two questions. The first question is regarding my choice to pursue an academic-research career vs. a much more lucrative clinical career. This question is mainly asked by my family including my children. It is frequently a difficult question to answer but I can trace my desire to pursue a research interest in psychiatry to a specific incident. While an intern at Cairo University Faculty of Medicine (Giza Egypt) I was responsible for one of the outpatient clinics. One morning I had a family bring their 16-year-old daughter for an evaluation. When their turn came, they were ushered in by the assistant. There was the father, mother, and the daughter (the identified patient). For all intents and purposes the family looked like a stable middle-class family. After being seated, I asked the usual opening question of "what brings you to the clinic today?" Upon me asking the question the mother asked the father to leave the room. Once the father left the room the mother asked the daughter to disrobe. What I saw at that moment imprinted in my memory for rest of my life and seriously impacted my career. The girl (who is well educated and by all indications smart) had cuts allover her arms and legs in addition to scars from cigarette burns on her abdomen. She has attempted *suicide* multiple times. She had all the manifestations that are needed to earn her the diagnosis of *Borderline Personality Disorder.* I spent most of the remaining appointment time asking routine historical questions then performed a standard mental status examination. During the intervening week I read all what I could find about this disorder. My dissatisfaction was great. The main thing I learned was that it was likely that the father has abused her, and that treatment consisted mainly of vaguely defined therapies. Cure was not assured by any means. This to me was triple bad news that I needed to convey to the family. In the next visit I met with the father first and confronted him with the prevailing theories. He absolutely denied any wrongdoing. He was credible. I then interviewed the mother also separately. She also denied any possibility that the father has abused his daughter, so did the daughter also when interviewed both separately and in her mother's presence. They were all credible, but the literature was not. I concluded that this patient was not simply seeking attention but that she was suffering from an ailment that as of that time (and sadly till today) is poorly understood. There was nothing for me to offer this family. My further reading added much more evidence to my conclusion that our knowledge of what we do in psychiatry remains severely minimal and that much more research was absolutely necessary. This sounded to me as a worthwhile goal for my career. Furthermore, academic careers have their own rewards. Constant interacting with younger individuals like students and residents is invigorating. Life in pursuit of new knowledge does not allow for boredom. The thrill of getting funded to do your proposed research is a serious ego booster but of course is surpassed when one publishes his/her research in respected journals. Conferences and other scientific gatherings make for other intellectually stimulating enjoyable experiences. Finally, a significant measure of recognition as well as life-time job security are achieved once a faculty member is awarded tenure by his/her institution. While these answers did little to satisfy my family members, they indeed were quite satisfying for me to keep pursuing the goals I set for myself.

The other question was regarding my motivation for writing this book. Having practiced both Psychiatry and Neurology and influenced by the teachings of Humanism I felt I had a unique perspective. Simply stated I wanted to share and archive my opinion regarding the current day practice of Psychiatry and underscore my optimism for the future of the field. If a single idea, from the many listed throughout the book, found its way to implementation I would indeed be quite contented with my entire career.

REFERENCES

ACGME, 2007. *ACGME program requirements for graduate medical education in child and adolescent psychiatry.* www.acgme.org/acWebsite/RRC_400/400_prIndex.asp.

AGREE Collaboration: Development and validation of an international appraisal instrument for assessing the quality of clinical practice guidelines: the AGREE project. *Qual Saf Health Care* 2003;12:18-23.

Allen Frances, Allen. 2013. *Saving Normal: An insider revolt against out of control psychiatric diagnosis, DSM-5, big pharma and the medicalization of ordinary life.* William Morrow/Harper Collins Publishers; 2013.

Allom, V., Mullan, B., Hagger, M. 2016. Does inhibitory control training improve health behaviour? A meta-analysis, *Health Psychology Review*, 10:2, 168-186. doi: 10.1080/17437199.2015.1051078. (Allom et al, 2016).

Amad, A., Ramoz, N., Thomas, P., Jardi, R., and Gorwood, P. Genetics of borderline personality disorder: systematic review and proposal of an integrative model. *Neurosci Biobehav Rev.* 2014 Mar;40:6-19. doi: 10.1016/j.neubiorev.2014.01.003. Epub 2014 Jan 20.

American Psychiatric Association: *Diagnostic and Statistical Manual of Mental Disorders, Fourth Edition.* Washington DC, American Psychiatric Association, 1994.

Andrulonis, P. A., Glueck, B. C., Stroebel, C. F. Borderline personality subcategories. *J Nerv Ment Dis* 1982; 170:670.

Arfken, C. L., Joseph, A., Sandhu, G. R., Rhoers, T., Douglass, A., B., and Boutros, N. N. The status of sleep abnormalities as a diagnostic test for major depressive disorder. *J of Affective Disorders*, 156:36-45, 2014.

Balsters, J. H., Mantini, D., Apps, M. A., Eickhoff, S. B., and Wenderoth, N. Connectivity-based parcellation increases network detection sensitivity in resting state fMRI: An investigation into the cingulate cortex in autism. *Neuroimage Clin*. 2016 Mar 25.

Barnes, J. C., Boutwell, B. B. A demonstration of the generalizability of twin-based research on antisocial behavior. *Behav Genet*. 2013 Mar;43(2):120-31. doi: 10.1007/s10519-012-9580-8. Epub 2012 Dec 29.

Bassiouni, M. 1966. The Right of the Mentally Ill to Cure and Treatment: Medical Due Process. DePaul University Library. *DePaul Law Review,* 15(4).

Blake, P. Y., Pincus, J. H., Buckner, C. Neurologic abnormalities in murderers. *Neurology* 45; 1641-1647, 1995.

Boelhouwer, C., Henry, C., Glueck, B. C. Jr. Positive spiking: a double blind controlled study on its significance in behavior disorders, both diagnostically and therapeutically. *Am J Psychiatry* 125; 473-480, 1968.

Boudreaux, J. M., Thompson, J. W Jr. Maternal-Fetal Rights and Substance Abuse: Gestation without Representation. *J Am Acad Psychiatry Law*. 2015 Jun;43(2):137-40.

Boutros N. N. (Ed). *International Psychiatry and Behavioral Neurosciences, Year Book Volume II.* Nova Science Publishers. January 2013; ISBN: 978-1-62257-566-4.

Boutros, A., Kang, S. S., Boutros, N. N. A Cyclical Path to Recovery: Calling into question the wisdom of Incarceration after Restoration.

International Journal of Law and Psychiatry. 2018 Mar - Apr; 57:100-105. doi: 10.1016/j.ijlp.2018.01.007. Epub 2018 Feb 10. Review. PMID: 29548496.

Boutros, N. N., Arfken, C., Galderisi, S. The status of EEG abnormality as a diagnostic test for schizophrenia. *Schizophr Res* 2008; 99:225-37.

Boutros, N. N., Bower, S., Wang, J., Urfy, M. Z., Loeb, J. A. Epilepsy spectrum disorders: A concept in need of validation or refutation. *Med Hypotheses*. 2015 Nov; 85(5):656-63.

Boutros, N. N., Bowers, M. B. Jr, Quinlan, D. Chronological association between increases in drug abuse and psychosis in Connecticut state hospitals. *J Neuropsychiatry and Clinical Neurosciences* 10 (1):48-54, 1998.

Boutros, N. N., Galloway, P. M., Philgren, E. M. Stimulants and Psychosis. In *Secondary Schizophrenia: Organic Syndromes of schizophrenia: drugs and schizophrenia-like psychoses*. Keshavan M & Sachdev P (Eds). Cambridge University Press, pp127-140, 2009.

Boutros, N. N., Gruber, N., Radentz, S. An account of patient population on a state hospital neuropsychiatry unit. *Integrative Psychiatry,* 7;2:126-127, 1991.

Boutros, N. N., Mucci, A., Vignapiano, A., Galderisi, S. Electrophysiological aberrations associated with negative symptoms in schizophrenia. In “Electrophysiology and Psychophysiology in Psychiatry and Psychopharmacology” volume of *Current Topics in Behavioral Neurosciences.* Kumari V, Boutros NN, Bob P Editors. Current Topics in Behavioral Neurosciences” (Series Editors Profs. Charles Marsden, Bart Ellenbroek and Mark Geyer). Springer Publisher, 2014; pp 129-156.

Boutros, N., Bowers, M. Jr. Substance induced psychotic disorder. *Journal of Neuropsychiatry and Clinical Neurosciences*. 1996;8 (3) pp 262-269.

Brinkley, J. R., Beitman, B. D., Freidel, R. O. Low dose neuroleptic regimen in the treatment of borderline patients. *Arch Gen Psychiatry* 36:319–326, 1979.

Brites, D., Fernandes, A. Bilirubin-induced neural impairment: a special focus on myelination, age-related windows of susceptibility and associated co-morbidities. *Semin Fetal Neonatal Med.* 2015 Feb;20(1):14-9. doi: 10.1016/j.siny.2014.12.002. Epub 2014 Dec 19.

Bruns, D. 2003. The STARD initiative and the reporting of studies of diagnostic accuracy. *Clin Chem* 2003; 49:19-20.

Bussuyt, P. M., Reitsma, J. B., Bruns, D. E. Towards complete and accurate reporting of studies of diagnostic accuracy: the STARD initiative. *Clin Chem* 2003; 49:1-6.

Campanella, S. 2016. Neurocognitive rehabilitation for addiction medicine: From neurophysiological markers to cognitive rehabilitation and relapse prevention. *Prog Brain Res.* 2016;224:85-103. doi: 10.1016/bs.pbr.2015.07.014. PMID: 2682235. (Campanella 2016).

Carpenter, W. T., Gunderson, J. G. Five-year follow-up comparison Neurology 45; 1641-1647, 1995 of borderline and schizophrenia patients. *Compr Psychiatry* 18:567–571, 1977.

Cerdá, M., Wall, M., Keyes, K. M., Galea, S., and Hasin, D. 2016. *Medical marijuana laws in 50 states; investigating the relationship between state legalization of medical marijuana and marijuana use, abuse and dependence.* doi: http://dx.doi.org/10.1016/ j.drugalcdep.2011.06.011. (Cerdá et al, 2016).

Clark, D. L., Boutros, N. N., Mendez, F. M. *Brain and Behavior: An Introduction to Behavioral Neuroanatomy.* Fourth Edition; Cambridge University Press, 2018.

Coccaro, E. F., Kavoussi, J. R. Biological and pharmacologicalaspectsof borderline personality disorder. *Hosp Comm Psychiatry* 1991; 42:1029–1033.

Coccaro, E. F., Sripada, C. S., Yanowitch, R. N., and Phan, K. L. Corticolimbic function in impulsive aggressive behavior. *Biol Psychiatry.* 2011 Jun 15;69(12):1153-9. doi: 10.1016/j.biopsych. 2011.02.032. Epub 2011 May 4.

Cowdry, R. W., Gardner, D. L. Pharmacotherapy of borderline personality disorder. *Arch Gen Psychiatry* 45:111–119, 1988.

Davies, R. K. 1979. Incest: some neuropsychiatric findings. *Int J Psychiatry Med* 9:117-121, 1979.

De Wilde, O. M., Bour, L. J., Dingemans, P. M. P300 deficits are present in young first episode patients with schizophrenia and not in their healthy young siblings. *Clin Neurophysiol* 2008; 119:2721-6.

Degenhardt, L., et al. (88 collaborators). Estimating treatment coverage for people with substance use disorders: an analysis of data from the World Mental Health Surveys. *World Psychiatry.* 2017 Oct;16(3):299-307. doi: 10.1002/wps.20457.

DSM-IV Sourcebook, Vol. 3. 1st Edition. by American Psychiatric Association Task Force on Dsm-IV (Author), Thomas A. Widiger (Editor), Allen J. Frances (Editor), Harold Alan Pincus (Editor), Ruth Ross (Editor), Michael B. First (Editor), Wendy Wakefield Davis (Editor) & 4 more. ISBN-13: 978-0890420737.

Duncan, N. W., Hayes, D. J., Wiebking, C., Tiret, B., Pietruska, K., Chen, D. Q., Rainville, P, Marjanska, M., Ayad, O., Doyan, J., Hodaie, M., and Northoff, G. Negative childhood experiences alters a prefrontal-insular-motor cortical network in healthy adults: a preliminary multimodal rsfMRI, fMRI, MRS, dMRI study. *Human Brain Mapping* 36(11):4622-4637, 2015.

Eaton, K., Ohan, J. L., Stritzke, W. G., K., Courtauld, H. M., and Corrigan, P. W. Mothers' Decisions to Disclose or Conceal Their Child's Mental Health Disorder. *Qual Health Res.* 2017 Sep;27(11):1628-1639. doi: 10.1177/1049732317697096. Epub 2017 Mar 20.

Fenwick, P. EEG studies, in *Epilepsy and Psychiatry*. Edited by Reynolds EH, Trimble MR. New York, Churchill-Livingstone, 1981.

Fleischman, P. Using independent mental health advocates. *Nursing Times* 111(45):22-24, 2015.

Ford, G., LaFranchi, S. H. Screening for congenital hypothyroidism: a worldwide view of strategies. *Best Pract Res Clin Endocrinol Metab.* 2014 Mar;28(2):175-87. doi: 10.1016/j.beem.2013.05.008. Epub 2013 Jun 18.

Frances, Allen. *Saving Normal: An insider revolt against out of control psychiatric diagnosis, DSM-5, big pharma and the medicalization of ordinary life.* William Morrow/Harper Collins Publishers; 2013.

Franklin, T. B., Mansuy, I. M. The involvement of epigenetic defects in mental retardation. *Neurobiol Learn Mem.* 2011 Jul;96(1):61-7. doi: 10.1016/j.nlm.2011.04.001. Epub 2011 Apr 28.

Gillberg, C., Steffenburg, S., Jakobsson, G. 1987. Neurobiological findings in 20 relatively gifted children with Kanner-type autism or Asperger syndrome. *Developmental Medicine & Child Neurology* 29(5):641-9.

Gjerde, L. C., Czajkowski, N., Roysamb, E., Ystrom, E., Tambs, K., Aggen, S. F., Orstavik, R. E., Kendler, K. S., Reichborn-Kjennerud, T., and Knudsen, G. P. Longitudinal, population-based twin study of avoidant and obsessive-compulsive personality disorder traits from early to middle adulthood. *Psychol Med.* 2015 Dec; 45(16):3539-48. doi: 10.1017/S0033291715001440. Epub 2015 Aug 14.

Gonzalez Vazquez, A. I., Seijo Ameneiros, N., Diz Del Valle, J. C., Lopez Fernandez, E., and Santed German, M. A. Revisiting the concept of severe mental illness: severity indicators and healthcare spending in psychotic, depressive and dissociative disorders. *J Ment Health.* 2017 Aug 10:1-7. doi: 10.1080/09638237.2017.1340615. [Epub ahead of print].

Greenwald, G. 2009. *Drug decriminalization in Portugal: Lessons for creating fair and successful drug policies.* The CATO Institute. (Greenwald 2009).

Groce, N., Challenger, E., Berman-Bieler, R., Farkas, A., Yilmaz, N., Schultink, W., Clark, D., Kaplan, C., and Kerac, M. Malnutrition and disability: unexplored opportunities for collaboration. *Paediatr Int Child Health.* 2014 Nov;34(4):308-14. doi: 10.1179/2046905 514Y.0000000156. Epub 2014 Oct 13.

Grosse, S. D., Van Vliet, G. Prevention of intellectual disability through screening for congenital hypothyroidism: how much and at what level? *Arch Dis Child.* 2011 Apr;96(4):374-9. doi: 10.1136/adc. 2010.190280. Epub 2011 Jan 17.

Gunderson, J. G., Kolb, J. E., Austin, V. The diagnostic interview for borderline patients. *Am J Psychiatry* 1981; 138:896–903.

Harden, B. J., Buhler, A., Parra, L. J. Maltreatment in infancy: A developmental Perspective on prevention and intervention. *Trauma Violence Abuse* 17(4):366-386, 2016.

Harper, M. A., Morris, M., Bleyerveld, J. The significance of an abnormal EEG in psychopathic personalities. *Aus. NZ J Psychiatry* 6;215-224, 1972.

Harrington, Anne. *Mind Fixers; Psychiatry's Troubled Search for the Biology of mental Illness*. W. W. Norton & Company, New York/London. 2019. ISBN: 978-1-324-00197-3.

Hill, D., Watterson, D. Electroencephalographic studies of psychopathic personalities. *J Neurol Psychiat* 5:47-65, 1942.

Hollister, L. E., Boutros, N. N. Clinical use of CT and MR scans in psychiatric patients. *J Psychiatr Neurosci* 16;4:194-198, 1991.

Howard, R. C. The clinical EEG and personality in mentally abnormal offenders. *Psychol Med* 14; 569-580, 1984.

Howson, C. P., Kennedy, E. T., Horwitz, A., editors. Prevention of Micronutrient Deficiencies: Tools for Policymakers and Public Health Workers. *Institute of Medicine (US) Committee on Micronutrient Deficiencies*; Washington (DC): National Academies Press (US); 1998.

Iofrida, C., Palumbo, S., Pelligrini, S. Molecular genetics and antisocial behavior: where do we stand? *Exp Biol Med* (Maywood). 2014 Nov;239(11):1514-23. doi: 10.1177/1535370214529508. Epub 2014 Apr 24.

Ito, Y., Teicher, M. H., Glod, C. A. Preliminary evidence for aberrant cortical development in abused children: a quantitative EEG study. *J Neuropsychiatr Clin Neurosci* 1998; 10:298–307

Jang, K. L. The University of British Columbia Twin Project: still figuring out what personality is and does. *Twin Res Hum Genet.* 16(1):70-72, 2013. doi: 10.1017/thg.2012.70. Epub 2012 Oct 9.

Jeon, Y. W., Polich, J. Meta-analysis of P300 and schizophrenia: patients, paradigms, and practical implications. *Psychophysiology* 2003; 40:684-701.

Kaldoja, M.L., Saard, M., Lange, K., Raud, T., Teeveer, O.K., and Kolk, A. Neuropsychological benefits of computer-assisted cognitive rehabilitation (using FORAMENRehab program) in children with mild traumatic brain injury or partial epilepsy: A pilot study. *J Pediatr Rehabil Med*. 2015;8(4):271-83. doi: 10.3233/PRM-150346.

Kazdin, A. E., Durbin, K. A. Predictors of child-therapist alliance in cognitive-behavioral treatment of children referred for oppositional and antisocial behavior. *Psychotherapy (Chic).* 2012 Jun; 49(2):202-17. doi: 10.1037/a0027933. PMID: 22642524.

Korzekwa, M., Links, P., Steiner, M. Biological markers in borderline personality disorder: new perspectives. *Can J Psychiatry* 1993; 38(suppl 1):S11–S15.

Kosten, T. A., Rounsaville, B. J. Sensitivity of psychiatric diagnosis based on the best estimate procedure. *Am J Psychiatry* 1992; 149:1225-7.

Kurtz, Paul. 2000. *The Humanist Manifesto 2000*. Prometheus Books; Amherst, New York. (Kurtz, 2000).

Lambert, B. L., Bann, C. M., Bauer, C. R., Shankaran, S., Bada, H. S., Lester, B. M., Whitaker, T. M., LaGasse, L. L., Hammond, J., and Higgins, R. D. Risk-taking behavior among adolescents with prenatal drug exposure and extrauterine environmental adversity. *J Dev Behav Pediatr*. 2013 Nov-Dec;34(9):669-79. doi: 10.1097/01.DBP.000043 7726.16588.e2.

Lange, S., Probst, C., Gmel, G., Rehm, J., Burd, L., and Popova, S. Global Prevalence of Fetal Alcohol Spectrum Disorder Among Children and Youth: A Systematic Review and Meta-analysis. *JAMA Pediatr*. 2017 Oct 1;171(10):948-956.

Legal, Inc. US. "USLegal." *Dusky Standard Law and Legal Definition* | USLegal, Inc., US Legal, 1997, definitions.uslegal.com/d/dusky-standard/.

Lishman, W. A. 1978. *Organic Psychiatry: The psychological Consequences of Cerebral Disorders*. First Edition, Blackwell Scientific publications, Boston.

Lishman, W. A. 1987. *Organic Psychiatry: The psychological Consequences of Cerebral Disorders*. Second Edition, Blackwell Scientific publications, Boston.

Marshall, D. F., Passarotti, M., Ryan, K. A., Kamali, M., Saunders, E, F., Pester, B., McInnis, M. G., Langenecker, S. A. Deficient inhibitory control as an outcome of childhood trauma. *Psychiatric Research* 235:7-12, 2016.

Mason, E., McDougall, L., Lawn, J. E., Gupta, A., Cleason, M., Pillay, Y., Presern, M., Lukong, M. B., Mann, G., Wijnroks, M., Azad, K., Taylor, K., Beattie, A., Bhutta, Z. A., and Chopra, M. Lancet Every Newborn Study Group; Every Newborn Steering Committee. From evidence to action to deliver a healthy start for the next generation. *Lancet.* 384(9941):455-467, 2014. doi: 10.1016/S0140-6736(14)60750-9. Epub 2014 May 19.

McGlashan, T. H. The Chestnut Lodge follow-up study: III. Long term outcome of borderline personalities. *Arch Gen Psychiatry* 1986; 43:20–30.

Medford, N. 2014. Dissociative symptoms and epilepsy. *Epilepsy Behav* 30:10-13, 2014. doi: 10.1016/j.yebeh.2013.09.038.

Messner, E. Covert complex partial seizures in psychotherapy. *Am J Orthopsychiatry* 1986; 56:323–326.

Muller, R. J. Is there a neural basis for borderline splitting? *Compr Psychiatry* 1992; 33(2):92–104.

Musante, L., Ropers, H. H. Genetics of recessive cognitive disorders. *Trends Genet.* 2014 Jan;30(1):32-9. doi: 10.1016/j.tig.2013.09.008. Epub 2013 Oct 28.

Nelson, D., Boutros, N. The organic personality disorder. *Integrative Psychiatry* 1993;9(3-4):140-144.

Nelson, D., Boutros, N. The organic personality disorder. *Integrative Psychiatry* 1993;9(3-4):140-144.

Nursing Standard. Down's screening: the right to informed choice. *Nursing Standard* 31(7):27-27, 2016. https://doi.org/10.7748/ns.31.7.27.s24.

Okasha, A., Sadek, A., Abdel Moneim, S. Psychosocial and lectroencephalographic studies of Egyptian murderers. *Br J Psychiatry* 126;34-40, 1975.

Otto, Randy K. "Competency to Stand Trial." *Applied Psychology in Criminal Justice*, 2006, pp. 151–180. doi:10.1007/0-387-25227-4_6.

Perry, J. C. Depression in borderline personality disorder: lifetime prevalence at interview and longitudinal course of symptoms. *Am J Psychiatry* 1985; 142:15.

Petra, C. Interventions to reduce discrimination and stigma: the state of the art. *Soc Psychiatry Psychiatr Epidemiol* (2017) 52:249–258.

Poeppl, T. B., Eickhoff, S. B., Fox, P. T., Laird, A. R., Rupprecht, R., Langguth, B., and Bzdok, D. Connectivity and functional profiling of abnormal brain structures in pedophilia. *Hum Brain Mapp.* 2015 Jun; 36(6):2374-86.

Pope, H. G Jr., Jonas, J. M., Hudson, J. I. The validity of DSM-III borderline personality disorder. *Arch Gen Psychiatry* 1983; 40:23–30.

Prins, Seth Jacob, and Laura Draper. *Improving outcomes for people with mental illnesses under community corrections supervision: A guide to research-informed policy and practice.* New York, NY: Council of State Governments Justice Center, 2009.

Riley, T., Niedermeyer, E. Rage attacks and episodic violent behavior: electroencephalographic findings and general considerations. *Clin Electroencephalogr* 9;131-139, 1978.

Ropers, H. H. Genetics of early onset cognitive impairment. *Annu Rev Genomics Hum Genet.* 2010;11:161-87. doi: 10.1146/annurev-genom-082509-141640.

Rosenberg, H. J., Rosenberg, S. D., Williamson, P. D. A comparative study of trauma and posttraumatic stress disorder prevalence in epilepsy patients and psychogenic nonepileptic seizure patients. *Epilepsia* 2000; 41:447–452.

RSMO 552.010. (2016, August 28). *Section: 552.0010 Mental disease or defect defined.* Retrieved November 27, 2016, from http://www.moga.mo.gov/mostatutes/stathtml/55200000101.html

Ruth Dreifuss. The secret to fighting U.S. heroin epidemic. *CNN*, Updated 4:54 PM ET, Tue April 19, 2016 (dreifuss 2016).

Schmidt, P. M., Handleman, M.J., Bidder, T. G. Seizure disorder misdiagnosed as borderline syndrome. *Am J Psychiatry* 1989; 146:400–401.

Schroder, F. H., Hugosson, J., Roobol, M. J. Screening and prostate-cancer mortality in a randomized European study. *N Engl J Med* 2009; 360:1320-8.

Schulz, P. M., Soloff, P. H., Kelly, T. A family study of borderline subtypes. *J Personality Disorders* 1989; 3:217–229.

Shelley, B. P., Trimble, M. R., and Boutros, N. N. 2008. Electroencephalographic cerebral dysrhythmic abnormalities in the trinity of nonepileptic general population, neuropsychiatric, and neurobehavioral disorders. *J Neuropsychiatry Clin Neurosciences* 20(1):7-22.

Sithisarn, T., Granger, D. T., Bada, H. S. Consequences of prenatal substance use. *Int J Adolesc Med Health*. 2012;24(2):105-12. doi: 10.1515/ijamh.2012.016. Epub 2011 Nov 29.

Skeaff, S. A. Iodine deficiency in pregnancy: the effect on neurodevelopment in the child. *Nutrients.* 2011 Feb;3(2):265-73. doi: 10.3390/nu3020265. Epub 2011 Feb 18.

Soloff, P. H. Pharmacotherapy of borderline disorders. *Compr Psychiatry* 22:535–543, 1981.

Stafford-Clark, D., Taylor, F. H. Clinical and electroencephalographic studies of prisoners charged with murder. *J Neurol Neurosurg Psychiatry* 12;325-330, 949.

Stuart H. Reducing the stigma of mental illness. *Global Mental Health* 3, e17, pp 1-14, doi:10.1017/gmh.2016.11, 2016.

Stuart, H. Reducing the stigma of mental illness. *Global Mental Health* 3, e17, pp 1-14, doi:10.1017/gmh.2016.11, 2016.

Teicher, M. H., Anderson, S. L., Polcari, A., Anderson, C. M., Navalta, C. P., and Kim, D. M. The neurobiological consequences of early stress and childhood maltreatment. *Neurosci Biobehav Rev* 27:33-44, 2003.

Teicher, M. H., Dumont, N. L., Ito, Y., Vaituzis, C., Giedd, J. N., and Anderson, S. L. Preliminary evidence for abnormal cortical development in physically and sexually abused children using EEG coherence and MRI. *Ann N Y Acad Sci* 821:160-175, 1997.

Teicher, M. H., Ito, Y., Glod, C. A. Preliminary evidence for abnormal cortical development in physically and sexually abused children using EEG coherence and MRI. *Ann New York Acad Sci* 1997; 821:160–175.

Terraneo, A., Leggio, L., Saladini, M., Ermani, M., Bonci, A., and Gallimberti, L. 2016. Transcranial magnetic stimulation of dorsolateral prefrontal cortex reduces cocaine use: A pilot study. *Eur Neuropsychopharmacol.* 26(1):37-44. doi: 0.1016/j.euroneuro.2015. 11.011. Epub 2015 Dec 4. PMID: 26655188 (Terraneo et al, 2016).

Tuvblad, C., Fanti, K. A., Andershed, H., Colins, O. F., and Larsson, H. Psychopathic personality traits in 5 year old twins: the importance of genetic and shared environmental influences. *Eur Child Adolesc Psychiatry.* 2017 Apr;26(4):469-479. doi: 10.1007/s00787-016-0899-1. Epub 2016 Sep 28.

van Karnebeek, C. D., Stockler, S. Treatable inborn errors of metabolism causing intellectual disability: a systematic literature review. *Mol Genet Metab.* 2012 Mar;105(3):368-81. doi: 10.1016/j.ymgme. 2011.11.191. Epub 2011 Nov 30.

Van Praag, H. M. Over the mainstream: diagnostic requirements for biological psychiatric research. *Psychiatry Res* 1997;72:201-12.

Volkow, N. D., Koob, G. F., McLellan, A. T. 2016. Neurobiologic Advances from the Brain Disease Model of Addiction. *N Engl J Med.* 28;374(4):363-71. doi: 10.1056/NEJMra1511480. Review. (Volkow et al. 2016).

Vysohlid, J., Walton, H. J. 1990. Development of continuing medical education in Europe: a review. *Med Educ* 24: 406–412.

Waddell, C., Lipman, E., Offord, D. Conduct disorder: practice parameters for assessment, treatment, and prevention. *Can J Psychiatry*. 1999 Oct;44 Suppl 2:35S-40S.

Walton, H. J. 2001. Psychiatric Education and Training. In: Henn F., Sartorius N., Helmchen H., Lauter H. (eds) *Contemporary Psychiatry*. Springer, Berlin, Heidelberg.

Willging, C. E., Harkness, A., Israel, T., Ley, D., Hokanson, P. S., DeMaria, C., Joplin, A., and Smiley, V. Mixed-Method Assessment of a Pilot Peer Advocate Intervention for Rural Gender and Sexual Minorities. *Community Ment Health J*. 2017 Sep 16. doi: 10.1007/s10597-017-0168-x. [Epub ahead of print].

Wise, J. Second test for Down's Syndrome is recommended by the NHS. *BMJ* 352; 285, 2016. Doi:10,1136/bmj,.i285 pmid 26773062

Wong, M. T. H., Lumsden, J., Fenton, G. W. Electroencephalography, computed tomography and violence ratings of male patients in a maximum-security mental hospital. *Acta Psychiatr Scand* 90;97-101, 1994.

Zanarini, M. C., Williams, A. A., Lewis, R. E. Reported pathological childhood experiences associated with the development of borderline personality disorder. *Am J Psychiatry* 154:1101– 1106, 1997.

About the Author

Nash N. Boutros, MD is currently an Adjunct Professor of Psychiatry at RUSH-University Medical Center in Chicago. He also is director of Clinical Neurophysiology at the Neuroscience Center in Deerfield Illinois.

INDEX

A

B

C

D

E

F

G

H

I

M

N

O

P

R

S

T